PHYSICAL
PERFORMANCE
FITNESS AND DIET

Publication Number 1009

AMERICAN LECTURE SERIES®

A Monograph in

The BANNERSTONE DIVISION of
AMERICAN LECTURES IN ENVIRONMENTAL STUDIES

Edited by

CHARLES G. WILBER

Professor of Zoology
Colorado State University
Fort Collins, Colorado

PHYSICAL
PERFORMANCE
FITNESS AND DIET

By

D. R. YOUNG, B.S., M.A., Ph.D.

Research Scientist
NASA Ames Research Center
Moffett Field, California

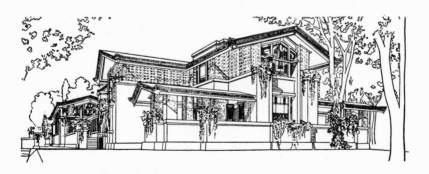

CHARLES   C   THOMAS   •   PUBLISHER
Springfield   •   Illinois   •   U.S.A.

Published and Distributed Throughout the World by
CHARLES C THOMAS • PUBLISHER
Bannerstone House
301-327 East Lawrence Avenue, Springfield, Illinois, U.S.A.

© *1977, by* CHARLES C THOMAS • PUBLISHER

ISBN 0-398-03642-X

Library of Congress Catalog Card Number: 76-56390

With THOMAS BOOKS *careful attention is given to all details of
manufacturing and design. It is the Publisher's desire to present books that
are satisfactory as to their physical qualities and artistic possibilities and
appropriate for their particular use.* THOMAS BOOKS *will be true to those
laws of quality that assure a good name and good will.*

Printed in the United States of America
R-1

Library of Congress Cataloging in Publication Data

Young, Donald R
    Physical performance, fitness, and diet.

    (American lecture series ; publication no. 1009)
    Bibliography: p.
    Includes index.
    1. Physical fitness--Nutritional aspects. 2. Sports
--Physiological aspects. 3. Work--Physiological
aspects. 4. Obesity--Complications and sequelae.
I. Title. [DNLM: 1. Exertion. 2. Physical fitness.
3. Nutrition. 4. Sport medicine. 5. Deficiency
diseases. WE103 Y69p]
RC1235.Y68   613.7   76-56390
ISBN 0-398-03642-X

FOREWORD

THE performance of mankind is determined by interaction of the individual with a host of environmental factors. Among these factors are physical, chemical, social, cultural, and biological components. "Influence is exerted by the various factors or elements as they exist as well as how they are perceived [by man]" (Trumbull, 1965).

Food is one of these environmental factors and its manipulation is one method readily available to improve human health, welfare, and fitness.

Food as an environmental factor for man has been rather widely neglected. It is only within the last few years that the critical role of food and nutrition in the welfare of the human species has become apparent. Extensive researches are now revealing that inadequate nutrition for a mother can wreck havoc on the offspring. Some of the disabilities as the result of inadequate maternal food are temporary. Unfortunately and alarmingly, some of these disabilities are permanent and result in a generation of offspring which are at a disadvantage, not because of their own genetics or actions but because their mother was exposed to a harmful environmental influence in the form of an inadequate diet (Handler, 1970; Dubos, 1968).

Newman (1962) has emphasized the key role of food as an environmental factor: ". . . nutritional stress in man has very strong ecological and cultural correlates. It should be equally apparent that the nutritional stresses that play such a potent role in human malaise must also impose their stamp on the forms and functions of many aspects of man's culture as well." The day to day ability of the individual human being to carry out, in an effective manner, his assigned tasks in the society in which he happens to live depends in a large part on the quality and the quantity of the food which is available to him. The

v

interrelationship of food, man, and environment is so close
that, although often overlooked, it cannot be denied.

Despite the fact that there is a critical need for a more precise
evaluation of food as an environmental factor related to physical fitness and the effectiveness of human performance,
Young in this book is forced to point out that "Our knowledge
today is based more or less on a data base available in 1958 to
1960." The fact remains that biological scientists are now faced
with a challenge to develop a total physiology of work capacity
as related to environmental variables. Among these variables
which must be given more adequate and more objective consideration is food — the fuel that permits the human machine to
operate at all.

The role of food and food elements in the overall welfare of
the individual human being is becoming more obvious as the
population ages and as various diseases peculiar to older persons begin to assert themselves. For example, the adverse action
of cholesterol as an environmental variable is obvious. Whether
cholesterol taken into the body as food is poisonous in terms of
circulatory health is still a matter of debate.

There does seem to be clear evidence, as an example, that
vitamin C, ascorbic acid, is a factor of importance in preventing pathological conditions which can be associated rather
directly with a chronic deficiency of vitamin C (Ginter, 1976). It
has been found by Ginter, for example, that there is a negative
correlation between the amount of vitamin C taken in by a
population and the standardized mortality ratios obtained from
cerebrovascular disease in different areas of England. Experiments have also demonstrated that vitamin C is remarkable in
its capacity to depress the concentration of plasma triglycerides:
These blood components seem to play a critical role in the
development of atherosclerosis. The studies with ascorbic acid,
then, emphasize the necessity for additional detailed experimental and epidemiological studies to ascertain more precisely
how ascorbic acid operates in the human body as well as what
levels are necessary to insure maximum operating capacity.

The role of exercise in the welfare of the human individual is
still a matter of some debate. It certainly seems apparent that

exercise by itself is not the key to life-long physical fitness. Certainly food as an environmental factor, no matter how it is manipulated, by itself cannot insure adequate levels of physical fitness.

Adaptation to caloric deficiency in man is known to occur (Grande, 1964): "The adaptation of the human body to caloric restriction involves the utilization of the body tissues as a source of chemical energy for the metabolism of the body and a reduction in the energy expenditure."

In order to use fat stores and cellular proteins extensively, significant changes in tissue enzyme activity occur as a metabolic adaptation. Secondly, energy expenditure is decreased by several physiological devices: Lowering of basal metabolic rate, decreased cost of physical activity, and lowered specific dynamic action. Most important in lowering the cost of activity is the voluntary reduction of activity (Taylor and Keys, 1950). Dubos (1968) contends that people reared in an environment where nutrition is quantitatively and qualitatively restricted adjust "by living less intensely." The relationship of food restriction with the resulting physiological adaptations to demanding physical performance in man is obscure. Is there a cross adaptation? Young presents information that suggests a potential close interrelationship of fasting, heavy exercise, and human adaptations. This complex problem deserves intensive and imaginative research. Part of the imaginative approach would be to insure more adequate and extensive data collected on the female of *Homo sapiens*.

Young refers to the serum growth hormone; he illustrates this substance with a model which is innovative and which presents material in a form which allows for exciting and new experimental approaches to the challenge of a total physiology of man with respect to significant environmental variables.

Dubos (1965) summarizes the critical role of food as an environmental factor with particular respect to protein deficiency. He says: "Protein deficiency and especially amino acid imbalance are responsible for high death rates among the young, poor physical development in the adults and a chronic illness that persists through life. This form of malnutrition (not necessarily undernutrition) probably constitutes the most important cause of disease in the underprivileged parts of the world."

Young devotes this monograph to the interrelationship of food and physical fitness; it seems appropriate to allude to the belief in the ancient world that diet could modify human behavior. Recent experiments suggest that this ancient belief does have a basis in fact. Ferrets, which ordinarily are rather vicious animals, become tame when fed a soft diet. Human mental activity and the ability to learn are clearly modified by the intake of protein and amino acid. Thus it is that the mental incapacity of children suffering from protein deficiency is so critical. This deficiency slows down mental development and indeed may result in permanent retardation of full mental abilities (Dubos, 1965).

A quarter of a century ago, Mitchel and Edman (1951) pointed out that an evaluation of human nutrition under stressful or nonstressful conditions through the use of experimental animals is no longer justified. There are both qualitative and quantitative differences between the rat (which is used so frequently in experimental biology) and man with respect to nutritional requirements. The extrapolation to man of information obtained on the albino rat is highly questionable. "Under climatic stress, the laboratory animal generally responds so differently, in kind or degree, from the human as to render comparison difficult" (Mitchel and Edman, 1951).

Many of the recommendations made in 1951 by Mitchel and Edman still need further study today. Young has brought out the present state of the art of the interrelationship of nutrition, physical activity, and physical fitness. It is obvious that this aspect of experimental biology of man requires further intensive study.

In all studies of human ecology is must be remembered that human performance is in the final stage based on psychological factors. These factors must be taken into account before one manipulates food in order to improve or change human activity for the better.

Dr. Charles G. Wilber
Editor

Literature Cited

Dubos, R.: *Man, medicine, and environment.* New York, NAL, 1968.

Dubos, R.: *Man adapting.* New Haven, Yale U Pr, 1965.

Ginter, E.: Vitamin C, blood cholesterol, and atherosclerosis. *American Laboratory 8(6):*21-29, 1976.

Grande, F.: Man under calorie deficiency. In Dill, D. B., Adolph, E. F., and Wilber, C. G. (Eds.): *Adaption to the Environment.* Washington, D.C., American Physiological Society, 1964.

Handler, P.: *Biology and the future of man.* New York, Oxford U Pr, 1970.

Mitchel, H. H. and Marjorie Edman: *Nutrition and Climatic Stress with Particular Reference to Man.* Springfield, Thomas, 1951.

Newman, M. T.: Ecology and nutritional stress in man. *American Anthropologist, 64:*22-33, 1962.

Taylor, H. L. and Keys, A.: Adaptation to caloric restriction. *Science, 112:*215-218, 1950.

Trumbull, R.: Environment modification for human performance. ONR Report ACR-105, Office of Naval Research, Washington, D.C., 1965.

PREFACE

THIS monograph deals principally with the relationships between diet, fitness, and physical work capacity. The extreme nutritional states considered are those associated with acute and chronic food deprivation as well as with obesity. Some attention is given to the effect of supplementation and modification of normal dietaries on work capacity. Within that context, the physiologic basis for dietary formulations is identified, and objective work performance is evaluated in terms of the responses to treadmill exercise or comparable stress tests.

Since the experimental and theoretical basis for providing nutrients for the support of physical work is based somewhat upon the metabolic responses to exercise, attention is given to current concepts regarding the metabolic events associated with work performance and in particular to carbohydrate and fat metabolism and their regulation by hormones. The approach taken has been to review the literature and to delineate the large grey areas where knowledge is incomplete, and also to discuss in some detail selected research studies that either have advanced knowledge or illustrate the breadth of the problems that researchers must address. This review covers principally human studies. Occasional references are made to animal research which have contributed to knowledge of the subject or which bring into sharp focus contrasting species responses.

Fitness and exercise programs for the maintenance of general health status have gained in popularity during the past fifteen to twenty years. This concept is reviewed briefly and some of the difficulties encountered in fitness programs are evaluated from an orthopedic point of view.

The final portion of the monograph summarizes and draws together the significance of the findings for the understanding of nutrition and performance. Overall, this monograph attempts to demonstrate the interdisciplinary nature of researches on diet, fitness, and performance, and also is an attempt to share with other life scientists and with graduate students the various biological disciplines employed in the studies.

CONTENTS

PHYSICAL
PERFORMANCE
FITNESS AND DIET

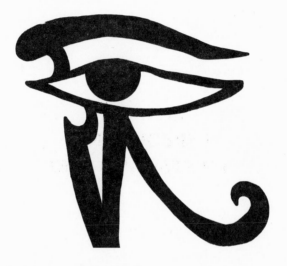

An Egyptian representation of the eye of Horus, the Sun God — sometimes called UDJAT . . . for the ancients it was a symbol of health.

Chapter 1

INTRODUCTION

SOME time has elapsed since the critical evaluation of the literature on diet and performance by Keys.[1] That extensive summary reviewed the earlier literature on dietetics and nutritional studies, and evaluated the findings in terms of the dominant concepts relevant to work performance and physical fitness in general. On the basis of Keys' review of in excess of 400 reports which claimed practical effects of various dietary components on performance along with an indication of the theoretical basis, the conclusions that emerge are as follows: (1) Total deprivation of food or water has the most obvious and dramatic effect on performance capacity; (2) for limited periods of time the effect on performance of vitamin, mineral, and general dietary imbalance may be of small consequence; and (3) performance will remain stable during moderate dietary variations, provided that the caloric needs are not too far from being satisfied and that the balance of fats, proteins, and carbohydrates is not too drastically and abruptly altered.

Although the early literature provides a firm data base for the formulation of theory and testing concepts regarding diet and performance, significant improvements in measurement and evaluation techniques, increased awareness as well as greater public health concern have had a major impact on the science of fitness and performance evaluation. Indeed, recent increased public concern for fitness in relationship to health has been expressed extensively through the self-prescription of exercise regimes on the one hand, and the intake of special and in some cases unusual diets on the other hand.

With the realization in the 1950's that cardiovascular disease and obesity were reaching epidemic proportions in the population, new relationships were sought between diet and performance on the one hand, and general health status on the other hand, with the emphasis on therapeutics and the intervention and prevention of disease. During that period, fewer publications were evident relating specific dietary components to performance and physical fitness or attempting to improve performance capacity through special dietary supplements; the available literature dealt largely with the development of minimum feeding concepts for survival-type situations as well as the nutrition of athletes. However, during that general period, there were significant breakthroughs in methodologies for the measurement of circulating levels of several hormones and also general acceptance and usage of radioisotope techniques for the measurement of lipid and carbohydrate metabolism in man. For the fundamental researcher, those provided the means for detailed investigations of the responses to exercise as well as to diet with the promise of uncovering the myriad of control and regulatory systems associated with body adjustments and altered physiologic states. By the early 1970s certain opinions appeared to emerge from a large and frequently controversial body of data relevant to diet, exercise, and health. Some of these concepts and points of view follow:

With regard to physical fitness achieved through exercise, it was for many years considered axiomatic that general health, leadership qualities, quality and life style, and even longevity were closely associated with a high level of fitness. During the past fifteen years that concept was examined in considerable detail in relationship to ischemic heart disease. Whereas exercise tests are of proven value in the assessment and diagnosis of diseases of the heart, clear scientific data in support of the contention that exercise and physical fitness can prevent myocardial infarction, for example, are meager. Naughton[2] cites very preliminary evidence suggesting that regular physical activity enhances the survival rate following myocardial infarction. But this author is aware of only one report[3] which demonstrates that progressive physical conditioning exercises raise the threshold for and reduce the frequency of premature ventricular complexes induced by physical stress tests. Some of the problems associated with epidemiological studies and controlled exercise trials for the prevention of coronary heart disease were reviewed by Taylor et al.[4] The sheer magnitude of the research requirements for the demonstration statistically of exercise prevention is staggering. It has been estimated that a five-year study with 30,000 men beyond the age of forty with diagnosed risk factors would be required in order to determine whether or not exercise intervention significantly modifies mortality and morbidity.[5] Additional considerations add to the complexity and magnitude of the test requirements. For example, if the distribution function of the incidence of heart disease is approximately "normal" or Gaussian, progressive time- and age-related physiologic deterioration is to be expected; therefore tests on young men also would be rewarding in order to elucidate the time-history and course of events associated with deterioration and failure characteristics. On the other hand, for a nominal age range in younger men, the probability of heart disease may be proportional only to the interval of time studied and independent of the age of the subject. The principle underlying that type of exponential reliability is one of chance or random failure for the age group considered. In a complex biological system this approach may be warranted due to variable changes in a multiplicity of physiologic systems, environmental conditions, and other predisposing factors. Exercise intervention studies in young men, therefore, would also be rewarding to reveal various stress-intensity combinations and patterns which may produce apparently random failures in time. Such studies would probably require a larger population sample than cited above, as well as early and improved diagnosis. We are also cautioned that rigorously standardized exercise programs and criteria of fitness, rather than general health evaluations based upon occupational activity levels, are required for the demonstration of effectiveness.

In another related area of concern, a relationship between cardiovascular disease and excessive body weight is suspected. Since exercise is believed to be of value for body weight management and control, it follows therefore that exercise could be of value in lowering the incidence of heart disease.

Although Mann[6] has reminded us that uncomplicated obesity (up to 35% body fat content) might be best dealt with and controlled through calorie management involving both physical exercise and reasonable menu planning, to date there is no clear relationship between moderate overweight and cardiovascular status. In the Framingham Study,[7] for example, overweight (at least until it reached high proportions) was inconsequential as a risk factor for all forms of coronary heart disease. Similarly, in a study of the incidence of coronary heart disease in seven countries, Keys et al.[8] concluded that when the influences and contributions of hypercholesteremia and high blood pressure were extracted from the data, the relationship between obesity alone and heart disease was of questionable statistical significance.

On the other hand, the consequences of overweight in the pathogenesis of diabetes mellitus are firmly established, and the incidence of both juvenile and maturity-onset forms of the disease increases dramatically with excessive body weight.[9] To the extent that a planned exercise program may assist in body weight control and improvement in general metabolism,[10] it may be a useful adjunct in the treatment of maturity-onset diabetes, but may possibly be of lesser value in the management of the more brittle juvenile-type disease.

Briefly reviewing the factors associated with the first (diseases of the heart) and the eighth (diabetes mellitus) leading causes of death in the U.S.A., the demonstration of prevention through physical conditioning is unproven and indeed largely untested rigorously.

In view of the somewhat disappointing evidence and the failure to demonstrate systematic and unequivocal improvements in health status through exercise, one may question seriously the value of exercise in the life process. Again in the 1950s, attention was focused on the shortcomings of physical fitness in the American population associated apparently with sedentary living habits more than to aging or other factors. In the opinion of some, the vitality and growth of a civilization could be related to fitness and the resistance of man, to the forces of nature, or against the onrush of a more vital enemy. That historical perspective may be questionable. Nevertheless, the value of a relatively high state of physical conditioning is evident in athletes, certain occupational groupings, the Armed

Forces, and a large and diverse group of sports enthusiasts for whom fitness is a requisite for performance capability. It is interesting to speculate on the advantages of exercise conditioning in a population which has no special job or avocation-related fitness requirements. Attainment of a moderate level of physical fitness may be related to cosmetic effects, to social acceptance, ego satisfaction, self-esteem, and a sense of self-fulfillment which are legitimate and valid goals in life. To some people, exercise is an important pattern integrated into a life style. It makes them sleep better and releases hostilities. They feel better and are more capable of being productive in their particular environments. No other defense of exercise need be sought.

With regard to the relationships between nutrition and fitness, it has been amply demonstrated that poor performance and easy fatigue are characteristics of frank deficiencies of many major dietary components. During acute periods of calorie restriction, diminished levels of the blood sugar, acidosis, and dehydration appear to be the dominant metabolic factors responsible for a diminished tolerance for physical work.[11] In chronic undernutrition, degraded levels of performance and personality changes[12] may ultimately be related to tissue enzyme changes.[13]

Mayer and Bullen[14] have summarized the state of knowledge with regard to the nutrition of athletes. During training, the intake of three balanced meals a day is recommended, with a moderate margin of excess high-quality protein for an increase in muscle mass, and perhaps a higher than normal intake of thiamine and possibly the entire vitamin B complex. An adequate electrolyte and water balance is also important. For the period just prior to athletic contests, light carbohydrate meals and strongly sweetened tea are favored; bulky and spicy foods are to be avoided. Stimulants such as coffee may mitigate the sense and awareness of fatigue.

The obese individual combining low calorie diets or fasting with exercise in order to attain a desirable body weight also encounters nutrition-related performance problems. Fasting,[15] for example, produces significant electrolyte and water-balance changes with subsequent decreases in blood pressure, heart size, and occasionally postural hypotension. During exercise, ketosis would probably dominate the metabolic factors leading to easy fatigue and poor performance, and supplementation with glucose would be a logical treatment of the problem.

Minimal feeding concepts are important in survival-type situations which require a high level of physical performance, and also to the avid outdoor enthusiast who voluntarily withdraws from typical feeding patterns and food resupply channels. Placed in proper perspective, an adequate level of performance under those conditions is related to: (1) protection from the environment and medical aid when necessary, (2) adequate water and salt, and (3) supply of food. The type and quantity of food taken can clearly prevent ketosis, prevent excessive body water loss, and maintain the blood sugar level.

Finally, during the past twenty years a considerable emphasis has been placed upon therapeutic nutrition, particularly in relationship to type and quantity of dietary fat. A recent article[16] chronicles the development and self-prescription of a diet for the treatment of generalized atherosclerosis and angina. Spectacular claims are made for supplementation with vitamins C, E, and B complex, unsaturated oils, lecithin, and bone meal. Although the benefits claimed tend to be largely anecdotal, the report does emphasize those dietary factors which have been subject to rigorous investigations by the nutritionist and biochemist, while at the same time defining atherosclerosis as a deficiency disease. The concept that many of our "typical" diets are deficient is difficult if not impossible to prove; nevertheless, it is believed to be true by a significant portion of the society. Here, again, on the subject of fat metabolism, exercise is believed by some to be of value in lowering the level of blood lipids, particularly the circulating levels of triglycerides, and thus in conjunction with therapeutic diets to be beneficial for the prevention of ischemic heart disease.

During the past ten to twenty years, there has been a relative reduction in the number of controlled laboratory trials relating objective physical performance to diet. This is perhaps due to the failure of finding special "ergogenic" substances or feeding schedules beyond typical dietaries which are deemed to be adequate according to the National Research Council allowances. Also, greater concern for public health aspects has oriented the interest and direction of research towards population studies, sampling and surveys as a means for tracking large populations in time.

At the present time, to reiterate the large number of studies on nutrition and performance vis-à-vis Keys would probably serve little useful purpose, since those earlier reports attempted frequently to evaluate the effect of discrete dietary variables on performance capacity and fitness, whereas the more recent approaches have addressed the broader subject of health status in its relationship to general nutrition and physical fitness. Within this context, many studies of the responses to exercise and the evaluation of physiologic potential and metabolic ceilings were undertaken to uncover metabolic subtleties and details of mechanisms of action. Outstanding developments in exquisite analytical and measurement techniques for the evaluation of energy metabolism and hormonal interactions, in a number of cases, led to firmer statements and conclusions related to exercise effects distinct from dietary-induced responses. Studies of the relationships between diet and performance which historically required a multidisciplinary team now encompassed an even wider group of subspecialties in order to assure techniques, methodologies, and the interpretation and handling of data. Major studies were no longer conducted by a relatively small number of highly specialized laboratories; instead there was a proliferation of activity in a large number of research environments. This led to an avalanche of data in fast-moving fields, notably fat and carbohydrate metabolism. The fragmentation had the unfortunate effect of creating a very dispersive literature not too visible to the interested reader.

In view of the foregoing, it would appear desirable to summarize and evaluate the older literature in conjunction with the more recent findings. Rather than simply listing a compendium of facts, the attempt here is to include the experimental evidence leading to current concepts relevant to nutrition, performance, and fitness.

REFERENCES

1. Keys, A.: Physical performance in relationship to diet. *Fed Proc, 2*:164-187, 1943.
2. Naughton, J.: Can myocardial infarction be prevented? *Medical Digest, 17*:30-39, 1971.
3. Blackburn, H., Taylor, H. L., Hamrell, B., Buskirk, E., Nicholas, W. C., and Thorsen, R. D.: Premature ventricular complexes induced by stress testing. Their frequency and response to physical conditioning. *Am J Cardiology, 31*:441-449, 1973.
4. Taylor, H. L., Buskirk, E. R., and Remington, R. D.: Exercise in controlled trials of the prevention of coronary heart disease. *Fed Proc, 32*:1623-1627, 1973.
5. Buskirk, E. R.: Personal communication.
6. Mann, G. V.: Obesity, the nutritional spook. *Am J Public Health, 61*:1491-1498, 1972.
7. Kannel, W. B., LeBauer, E. J., Dawber, T. R., and McNamara, P. M.: Relation of body weight to development of coronary heart disease. *Circulation, 35*:734-747, 1967.
8. Keys, A., Aravanis, C., Blackburn, H. B., van Buchem, F. S. P., Buzina, R., Djordjevic, B. S., Dontas, A. S., Fidanza, F., Karvonen, M. J., Kimura, N., Lekos, D., Monti, M., Puddu, V., and Taylor, H. L.: Epidemiological studies related to coronary heart disease: Characteristics of men aged 40-59 in seven countries. *Acta Med Scand Suppl, 460*:392-426, 1966.
9. Diabetes Source Book, Public Health Service Publication No. 1168, U.S. Dept. of Health, Education, and Welfare, Washington, D.C., 1968, 80 pp.
10. Harger, B. S., Miller, J. B., and Thomas, J. C.: The caloric cost of running its impact on weight reduction. *JAMA, 228*:482-483, 1974.
11. Henschel, A., Taylor, H. L., and Keys, A.: Performance capacity in acute starvation with hard work. *J Appl Physiol, 6*:624-633, 1954.
12. Brozek, J.: Starvation and nutritional rehabilitation. A quantitative case study. *J Am Diet Assoc, 28*:917-926, 1952.
13. Knox, W. E., Auerbach, V. H., and Lin, E. C. C.: Enzymatic and metabolic adaptations in animals. *Physiol Rev, 36*:164-254, 1956.
14. Mayer, J. and Bullen, B.: Nutrition and athletic performance. *Physiol Rev, 40*:369-397, 1960.
15. Bloom, W. L.: To fast or exercise. *Am J Clin Nutrition, 21*:1475-1570, 1968.
16. Rinse, J.: Atherosclerosis, chemistry and nutrition: Some observations, experiences, and an hypothesis. *American Laboratory*, pp. 25-37, July 1973.

Chapter 2

PERFORMANCE CAPACITY
AND NUTRITURE

IT is widely accepted that a poor nutritional state is incompatible with a high working capacity, and it is generally agreed that the best nutrition supports a physiologic state in which nutritional factors are not limiting for human performance of all types. Climatic stresses impose particular nutrient requirements that warrant further exploration. For example, it seems clear that climatic stress modifies greatly the body's requirements for food energy, water, and sodium chloride. It is less certain that under conditions of excessive sweating the dietary requirements for calcium and iron lost in the sweat are increased; there is even less assurance that hypoxia induced by altitude increases the requirement for vitamins, particularly ascorbic acid and thiamine. In some cases climatic factors are reported to increase the desire for specific foods, for example, a hunger for fatty foods in a cold environment or for sweet foods at high altitude. In fact, it has been reported that appetite per se plays a significant role in acclimatization to cold environments. This belief derives a degree of circumstantial support from observations that diets in hot climates sometimes tend to be low in fats and high in carbohydrates.

Despite an abundance of suggestive data for special diets for climatic usage, in general, barring injury or disease, people remain fit and healthy in temperate environments, jungles, deserts, and frigid areas when their diets provide an abundance and variety of foods, a balanced regimen of 15 percent of calories from protein, 50 percent from carbohydrate, 35 percent from fat, and all known minerals, vitamins, and cofactors in *luxus* amounts. On the other hand, limitation of salt and water, decrease in caloric intake, marked departures in protein/

11

carbohydrate/fat ratios, and marked deviations of osmotic intake will be associated with measurable clinical and functional
deterioration which may reach dangerous levels.

Much of the knowledge of the relationship between diet and
exercise capacity has been obtained in controlled experiments
involving partial or total food withdrawal. Starvation is obvi-
ously the poorest nutritional state, and studies of that state
provide estimates of the time history of performance degrada-
tions in relationship to food intake, as well as a general assessment of the importance of specific nutrients. In this section,
effects of food deprivation are discussed from the standpoint of
the resulting physiological and biochemical distortions as well
as effects on physical performance; minimum feeding concepts
required to maintain performance are discussed with an emphasis on the physiologic basis for the dietary composition;
finally, performance in relationship to special dietary supplements is reviewed.

EFFECT OF FOOD DEPRIVATION

Bearing in mind that various factors are involved in nutritional deficiencies, what type of picture may be drawn of the
effects on performance and the course of events which may be
expected to occur as a deficient state develops? Current knowledge is inadequate to establish precisely the pattern of deterioration in fitness. However, for general guidance a chart was
developed by Johnson and is reproduced here as Table I. The
data relate to the responses expected in a hot, humid environment, and therefore emphasize the importance of salt and water
intake. Nevertheless, the ranking in order of importance is
considered to be generally appropriate; it can be seen that easy
fatigue and poor performance are among the earliest effects to
appear in working men exposed to a complete deficiency of an
essential nutrient. Some of the reported effects of food deprivation on the performance of laboratory animals are shown in
Table II. Here the picture is somewhat less consistent than
anticipated. First, most studies of volitional activity tend to
measure animal drives and the corresponding overt behavior

TABLE I

RATE OF ONSET OF DEFICIENCY SYNDROMES IN WORKING
MEN EXPOSED TO COMPLETE DEFICIENCY OF ONE OR
MORE OF THE IMPORTANT NUTRIENTS[a]

Nutrient	Time Before Earliest Effects on Performance Appear in Complete Deficiency	Deficiency Syndrome and End Result
Water	A few hours.	Easy fatigue, poor performance, eventual exhaustion of dehydration.
Calories	Two or three days.	Easy fatigue, poor performance.
Sodium Chloride	One to three days.	Easy fatigue, poor performance. Eventually, heat cramps.
Carbohydrate	Several days.	Easy fatigue, poor performance. Eventually, nutritional acidosis.
Vit. B Complex	One or two weeks.	Easy fatigue, poor performance. Eventually, one of the B-deficiencies, usually beri-beri.
Vitamin C	Several weeks.	Easy fatigue, poor performance. Eventually, scurvy.
Protein	Probably several weeks.	Late result, nutritional edema.
Vitamin A	Several months.	Earliest effects not known.
Fats	Many months.	Earliest effects not known.

[a]Johnson, R. E.: *Gastroenterology,* *1*:838, 1943.

rather than performance capacity; hence few conclusions can be drawn relative to the performance of a consistently motivated subject. Second, the biochemistry of food deprivation differs significantly in different species. For example, the dog is remarkably resistant to starvation ketosis and the rat is somewhat less sensitive than man. In the two studies of the effects of calorie deprivation cited in Table II, running capacity in the dog was not subject to the effects of ketosis and associated water loss, and tended to increase during five days of fasting. In contrast, the laboratory rat showed decrements in running capacity. The potential for developing suitable tests for the measurement of performance capacity of animals as a criterion of nutritional reliability has been examined in some detail.[1] This

EFFECT OF FOOD DEPRIVATION ON PERFORMANCE IN ANIMALS

Nutrient	Dietary Treatment	Animal	Activity	Effect on Activity*	Reference
A. Water	(1) Deprivation	Rat	Running**	+	a
B. Minerals	(1) Total deprivation	Rat	Running	+	b
	(2) Mg deprivation	Rat	Running	-	a
	(3) P or Fe deprivation	Rat	Learning	-	c
C. Calories	(1) Total deprivation (fasting)***	Rat	Enforced running	-	d
	(2) Total deprivation (fasting)	Dog	Enforced running	+	e
D. Fat	(1) 1 to 10% fat	Rat, mouse	Swimming at 37°C	0	f
	(2) 10% fat	Rat, mouse	Swimming at 20°C	-	f
	(3) 40% fat	Rat	Swimming at 32°C	+	g
E. Protein	(1) Protein restriction	Rat	Running	-	h
	(2) Protein deprivation	Rat	Learning	-	i
	(3) Lysine deprivation	Rat	Running	+	j
	(4) Supplementation with cystine or glutamic acid	Rat	Learning	0	k
F. Vitamins	Deprivation:				
	(1) Vitamin A	Rat	Learning	0	l
	(2) Thiamine				
	a. Acute	Rat	Running	+	m
	b. Chronic	Rat	Running	-	m
	c. Chronic	Mouse	Aggressiveness	0	n
	(3) Thiamine and riboflavin	Rat	Learning	-	o, p
	(4) Thiamine, riboflavin, and nicotinic acid	Rat	Running	0	q
	(5) B-Complex				
	a. Acute	Rat	Learning	-	r

G. Miscellaneous "Factors"	Rat	Running	-[s]	
b. Chronic Addition of:				
(1) Desiccated liver	Rat	Swimming at 20°C	+[t]	
(2) Wheat germ oil	Guinea pig	Swimming at 37°C	+[u]	

* + = increase in activity; - = decrease in activity; 0 = no change in activity.
** Spontaneous running unless otherwise indicated.
*** Decrease in running was influenced by the previous diet in the following order: Fat < carbohydrate < protein.

[a] Wald, G. and Jackson, B. Proc Natl Acad Sci, 30:255, 1944.
[b] Smith, P. K. and Smith, A. H. Abstr Proc Am Physiol Soc, 1934.
[c] Bernhardt, K. S. J Comp Psychol, 22:273, 1936.
[d] Samuels, L. T., Gilmore, R. C., and Reinecke, R. M. J Nutrition, 36:639, 1948.
[e] Young, D. R. J Appl Physiol, 14:1018, 1959.
[f] Ershoff, B. H. J Nutrition, 53:439, 1954.
[g] Sheer, B. T., Dorst, S., Codie, J. F., and Soule, D. F. Am J Physiol, 149:194, 1947.
[h] Slonaker, J. R. Am J Physiol, 96:577, 1931.
[i] Bernhardt, K. S. J Comp Psychol, 22:269, 1936.
[j] Bevan, W., Lewis, G. T., Bloom, W. T., and Abess, A. T. Am J Physiol, 163:104, 1950.
[k] Pilgrim, F. J., Zabarenko, L. M., and Patton, R. A. J Comp Physiol Psychol, 44:26, 1951.
[l] Bernhardt, K. S. J Comp Psychol, 22:269, 1936.
[m] Guerrant, N. B. and Deutcher, R. A. J Nutrition, 20:589, 1940.
[n] Beeman, E. A. and Allee, W. C. Physiol Zool, 18:195, 1945.
[o] Maurer, S. J Comp Psychol, 20:385, 1935.
[p] Maurer, S. J Comp Psychol, 20:309, 1935.
[q] Richter, C. P. and Barelare, B. Am J Physiol, 127:199, 1939.
[r] Bernhardt, K. S. and Herbert, R. J Comp Psychol, 24:263, 1937.
[s] Jakway, I. J Comp Psychol, 26:157, 1938.
[t] Ershoff, B. H. Proc Soc Exp Biol Med, 77:488, 1951.
[u] Ershoff, B. H. and Levin, E. Fed Proc, 14:431, 1955.

is an area of research where the selection of animals, standardization of test equipment, and environmental conditions (particularly light intensity and temperature) have a strong influence on the stability of performance estimates from one measuring period to another. Furthermore, care must be exercised to assure that the criteria or predictors of performance are relevant to the intent of the study. Test methods are desired which impose a measurable and recognized strain in animals and from which data can be interpreted by current clinical thought.

In human subjects, the effects of complete food deprivation and chronic semistarvation are similar in some aspects, e.g. a slowing of the heart rate and depression of metabolic rate. However, in complete starvation the sense of hunger frequently disappears in several days whereas in semistarvation it increases steadily. Ketosis, which is typical of starvation in man, does not occur in semistarvation as long as dietary carbohydrate is available. On the other hand, the edema which is characteristic of chronic semistarvation does not appear in complete food deprivation. During total food deprivation, physical performance decrements coincide with a 10 to 15 percent body weight loss and are associated with poor cardiovascular adjustments to physical work, loss of coordination, ketosis and occasional nausea, and dehydration and hyperthermia if water intake is restricted. In chronic semistarvation, poor physical performance is related to poor cardiovascular adjustments, and decreases in strength and coordination.

Decrement in performance and, indeed, survival are related to the extent of body weight loss during food deprivation. One experimental dog[2] is reported to have survived following a 65 percent body weight loss, although guinea pigs[3] and rats[4] usually die upon losing 35 to 50 percent of initial body weight. Human adults and young[5, 6] survive losses of 50 to 60 percent of initial body weight during chronic semistarvation, and these are probably within the range of the lethal limit. The rate of body weight loss is related to level of physical activity and trends of calorie imbalance. In two sedentary professional fasters, subjects S[7] and L,[8] 22 and 25 percent of body weight was lost during a thirty-one and forty-day fast, respectively. In subjects expending approximately 3200 kg Cal daily but consuming only 1570 kg Cal of a mixed diet, 23 percent of body weight was lost in twenty-four weeks.[9] In an earlier study with sedentary subjects,[10] reducing food intake from 2200 to 1600 kg Cal daily resulted in a 12.1 percent weight loss within eighty days. The rate of weight loss that may be expected to occur during food restriction is shown in Figure 1. For general guidance, a chart was prepared in the course of the Minnesota studies[11] estimating the extent of body weight loss in relationship to calorie deficit; this is reproduced here as Table III.

Several tissues contribute significantly to the loss of body weight observed during starvation. With regard to body protein, the urinary nitrogen excretion in man is relatively stable and within the range of 9 to 10 gms daily for a month or more

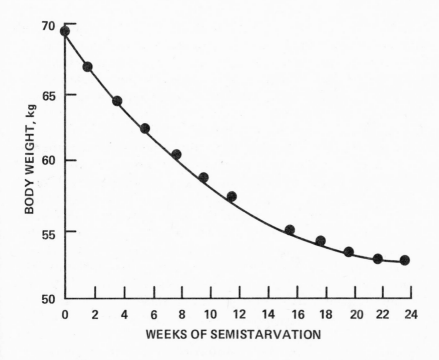

Figure 1. Body weight changes of physically active subjects on half rations. Body weight in kg is shown on the vertical scale; duration of food restriction is shown on the horizontal scale. (From Keys et al.: *The Biology of Human Starvation*, volume 1. Minneapolis, U of Minn Pr, 1950.)

TABLE III

BODY WEIGHT LOSS, AS PERCENTAGE OF INITIAL BODY WEIGHT

Duration	Calorie Intake As % Of Normal Balance						
(Months)	90	80	70	60	50	40	30
3	5	8	10	12	15	20	25
6	8	12	15	20	25	30	35
12 or more	10	15	20	25	30	35	40

ESTIMATES ARE BASED UPON REDUCED INTAKES WITH CALORIE VALUES EXPRESSED AS PERCENT OF INTAKE NEEDED FOR MAINTENANCE OF NORMAL WEIGHT.

From Keys et al.: *The Biology of Human Starvation,* volume 1. Minneapolis, U of Minn Pr, 1950.

during fasting. Animal tests of the effects of seven days of fasting[12, 13] show moderate to high protein losses from the liver, prostate, seminal vesicles, alimentary tract, kidneys, heart, muscle, and skin. Level of physical activity does not appear to modify rate of body protein losses during short periods of food deprivation; for example, the urinary nitrogen output in hard-working men during the course of a four- to five-day fast is substantially similar to that of inactive subjects.[14] Interestingly, functional thyroid tissue appears to be important for the breakdown and mobilization of body protein,[15] although in chronic semistarvation, the thyroid atrophies and the uptake of iodine by the gland is reduced more or less in proportion to the loss of body weight.[16, 17] The adrenal cortex, under the influence of the pituitary, plays an important role in the maintenance of the blood sugar through the enhancement of gluconeogenesis. Although the knowledge of mechanisms leading to adrenal changes during starvation is lacking, if the acutely deprived or semistarved laboratory rat is examined prior to the terminal phases, the adrenal is usually atrophied.[18, 19] At the same time, the pituitary atrophies[20, 21] and in consequence it has been suggested that adrenal atrophy is secondary to impaired function of the anterior pituitary gland rather than being a direct result of starvation.

But the possibility exists that alterations may occur in the selective secretion of various hormones from the pituitary during starvation. For example, total food deprivation causes an increase in cardiac glycogen in rabbits,[22] an effect which can be reproduced in the rat by the administration of growth hormone;[23] thus an increased secretion of growth hormone is suggested. Again, it was originally reported[24] that the pituitaries of chronically semistarved animals contained less gonadotrophic factors than those of normally fed controls; more recently it was shown that the gonadotrophic content of the pituitary of starved rats is greater on the basis of pituitary weight than in normal animals.[25] Therefore, in the overall, variations in the synthesis/release rates of the anterior pituitary hormones are implicated.

Other parameters in protein metabolism which have been measured are as follows: Plasma protein concentration remains relatively constant during acute starvation,[26] but decreases during chronic semistarvation to the point at which edema eventually appears. Plasma amino acids remain relatively constant;[27, 28] the concentration of blood urea usually shows a transitory increase during food deprivation but returns to normal values within several days;[29] blood level of uric acid is usually increased during food deprivation,[30, 31] and urinary excretion of urates is reduced.

Overall, the energy derived from protein metabolism contributes approximately 25 to 35 percent of total calorie requirements during fasting, and approximately 16 percent of calories during chronic semistarvation.

The blood glucose declines during the early phases of food deprivation and then stabilizes within the range of 60 to 72 mg percent for a prolonged period. The carbohydrate reserves are not a significant fraction of body mass and therefore have relatively little bearing on gross body weight changes. However, the maintenance of blood sugar is necessary to vital tissues (brain) which have an obligatory carbohydrate metabolism and is accomplished by endocrine mechanisms which enhance glucogenesis.[32, 33, 34]

Body fat disappears more rapidly than protein during starvation. In animals, when the body weight loss has reached 20 percent, as much as 55 to 75 percent of the body fat may have disappeared.[35] Approximately 50 percent is lost from the abdominal cavity and visceral organs, 30 percent from the subcutaneous depots, and 11 percent from muscle.[36] At death resulting from a 45 percent body weight loss, some 90 percent of initial body fat has been mobilized. The data on blood lipid changes occurring during the complete absence of food are variable. Keys et al.[37] reviewed the reported effects of five to fifty-seven days of total deprivation in healthy subjects. In some cases the total cholesterol concentration increases in the early phases and then decreases; in others there is an early decrease followed by a rise in concentration.

The reduction of body weight through loss of water, protein, and fat is somewhat offset by fluid shifts in the body. In animals which have starved until 45 percent of initial body weight had been lost, the water content per unit weight of muscle increased from a normal of 75.4 percent to 79.5 percent.[38] That relative increase and redistribution of body water content has also been reported in humans.[39, 40] During chronic semistarvation, the major part of the change in body water occurs in the extracellular space; during the twenty-four week Minnesota studies,[41] the thiocyanate space increased from a normal of 24 percent to 34 percent of contemporary body weight. Beattie et al.[42] reported a similar increase in a larger population subject to chronic undernutrition. During the Minnesota tests, the plasma volume per unit of body weight increased 41 percent while the extracellular fluid volume increased by 43 percent on the same basis. During acute starvation, the lack of edema suggests that the blood volume can be maintained within reasonable limits. However, in chronic semistarvation, especially on low protein diets, the body is unable to sustain that protection; indeed the intake of excessive water and sodium chloride can lead to a prompt increase in body weight and edema.[43]

The body mineral losses tend to be unremarkable. During complete food deprivation, the urinary excretion of sodium, potassium, and chloride is reduced. The serum concentrations of sodium, potassium, magnesium, calcium, and phosphorus show only minor fluctuations. In the early phases of food deprivation there is a moderate decline in serum chloride while the bicarbonate changes inversely with the extent and degree of ketosis. In the later phases of food deprivation, a substantial fall in serum chloride may be in part compensated by an increase in bicarbonate.[44] There is also a certain amount of decalcification of the skeletal system, and in chronic semistarvation the level of serum calcium declines.[45, 46]

No unequivocal evidence of vitamin deficiency has been reported during periods of total starvation. One explanation offered is that vitamins are supplied through the breakdown of body tissues.[47] It has been suggested that a high intake of vitamin C may aid in withstanding the debilitating effects of starvation.[48]

The biochemical distortions measured during food deprivation are considerable, yet the physiologic factors which impact on work performance capacity are relatively few and include: Hyperthermia, if water is restricted; low blood sugar and ketosis; and cardiorespiratory deconditioning.

MINIMUM FEEDING CONCEPTS

Planning menus and dietaries for minimal feeding concepts with the emphasis on the maintenance of physical fitness and work capacity is a considerable task. It is a subject about which much has been written and for which significant debate continues. The prior discussion of the effects of food deprivation shows the inevitability of performance decrements during starvation and suggests a general time history of deterioration in relationship to specific nutrient deficiencies as well as body weight loss. This constitutes physiologic evidence for the requirement for at least some food during periods of austerity when performance is at a premium. The critical factors in dietary planning are related to anticipated levels of energy expenditure, the feeding period, and distribution of calories; the need for water is important, e.g. hard work in a hot environment may raise the sweat losses to 10 *l*/day and work in a cold environment may increase sweat losses due largely to the insulating qualities of the protective clothing; the need for salt is important; the avoidance of acidosis is equally important. In addition, acceptability and palatability of the diet, stability in the absence of refrigeration, utility in packaging, and a requirement for a minimum of food preparation are other important considerations.

It is important at this point to review and evaluate briefly some of the indices of fitness believed to provide a rigorous assessment of performance capability and which, in part, provided the basis for performance evaluations in relationship to dietary austerity and minimal feeding concepts. These are

TABLE IV

EFFECT OF PHYSICAL FITNESS IN MAN ON
PHYSIOLOGIC RESPONSES TO WORK

Level of Activity	Index	Relative Change In Unfit Subjects*	Reference
A. At rest.	1. Pulse rate	+	a, b
B. Easy work that can be sustained in the steady state.	1. O_2 consumption	+	c
	2. CO_2 production	+	c
	3. R.Q.	+	d
	4. Ventilation	+	e, f
	5. Respiratory rate	+	e
	6. O_2 pulse	-	g
	7. Ventilatory efficiency	-	e
	8. Pulse rate	+	c, h
	9. Pulse rate deceleration after work	-	c, j
	10. Systolic pressure	+	h
	11. Rate of decline of systolic pressure after work	-	h
	12. Cardiac output — stroke volume	-	h, j
	13. Mechanical efficiency	-	c, h
	14. Blood lactate during work	+	k, j
C. Exhausting work that cannot be sustained in the steady state.	1. Duration	-	l, m, n
	2. Maximal O_2 uptake	-	o, p
	3. Maximal CO_2 production	-	o
	4. R.Q.	+	c
	5. Maximal ventilation	+	e

6. Ventilatory efficiency	-	d
7. O_2 pulse	-	g
8. Maximal pulse rate	+	g, p
9. Pulse rate deceleration after work	-	g, p
10. Systolic pressure	-	1
11. Rate of decline of blood pressure after work	-	1
12. Blood lactate at end of work	-	o
13. Blood sugar at end of work	-	q
14. O_2 debt	-	a, o

*+ or - refers to relative increase or decrease as compared to a physically fit subject.
[a]Knehr, C. A., Dill, D. B., and Neufeld, W. *Am J Physiol, 136*:148, 1942.
[b]Prosch, F. *Research Q, 4*:75, 1932.
[c]Dill, D. B., Talbot, J. H., and Edwards, H. T. *J Physiol, 69*:267, 1930.
[d]Steinhaus, A. H. *Physiol Rev, 13*:103, 1933.
[e]Briggs, H. *J Physiol, 54*:292, 1920.
[f]Taylor, C. *Am Physiol, 135*:27, 1941.
[g]Schneider, E. C. and Crampton, C. B. *Am J Physiol, 129*:165, 1940.
[h]Bock, A. V., Van Caulaert, C., Dill, D. B., Folling, A., and Hurxthal, L. M. *J Physiology, 66*:136, 1928.
[i]Dill, D. B. and Brouha, L. *Travail Humain, 5*:1, 1937.
[j]Dill, D. B. *Physiol Rev, 16*:263, 1936.
[k]Edwards, H. T., Brouha, L., and Johnson, R. E. *Travail Humain, 8*:1, 1940.
[l]Dawson, P. *The Physiology of Physical Education.* Baltimore, Baltimore Press, 1935.
[m]Schneider, E. C. *Physiology of Muscular Activity.* Philadelphia, W. B. Saunders, 1939.
[n]Bainbridge, F. A. *The Physiology of Muscular Exercise.* New York, Longmans Green, 1931.
[o]Robinson, S and Harmon, P. M. *Am J Physiol, 132*:757, 1941.
[p]Robinson, S., Edwards, H. T., and Dill, D. B. *Science, 85*:409, 1937.
[q]Robinson, S. *Arbeits Physiologie, 10*:251, 1938.

shown in Table IV with an emphasis on those factors which are related to physical endurance capacity. Several important criteria are brought out in this tabulation. For relatively short-term exhaustive work, the duration of effort is less in the unfit or deconditioned subject; the maximal O_2 uptake is less despite an increase in pulmonary ventilation rate, and the heart rate is higher, thus indicating a loss of cardiorespiratory fitness; blood pressure and heart rate are slow to decline following work, indicating a relative lack of compensatory homeostatic regulation; the oxygen debt and blood lactate are reduced, indicating some loss in anaerobic metabolic capacity. For easy to moderate work which can be sustained for a prolonged period, deconditioning and loss of fitness are dominated by a relative loss of physiologic economy and efficiency and therefore work is performed at a higher cost to the body. Thus, oxygen consumption increases as does the respiratory rate and heart rate; cardiac output stroke volume is reduced; and there is a greater tendency towards anaerobic metabolism with a corresponding increase in blood lactate.

In preliminary trials addressed to the subject of minimum food requirements, a series of detailed studies was undertaken by the Minnesota group[49, 50, 51] to evaluate the mechanisms of loss of fitness during food deprivation with unlimited water intake. In a five-day study, fit young subjects expended 2500 kg Cal daily, above and beyond the sedentary maintenance energy requirements, through sessions of treadmill walking. By the second day of fasting, work pulse rates were increased ten to fifteen beats/min and recovery heart rate was increased twenty beats/min, thus indicating a loss of cardiovascular reserve. The blood sugar declined 25 mg percent. The capability to perform short bouts of exhaustive running was impaired on the second day and continued to diminish until the fifth day. During daily sessions of treadmill walking, nausea and vomiting were experienced frequently and were associated with the ketosis. Strength remained stable, but speed of hand motion was reduced in parallel with the reduced level of blood sugar. Acidosis and dehydration were dominant factors responsible for the decreased performance capability.

The studies by Gamble[52] provided important guiding information relevant to body water conservation achieved through dietary means, and also some clues pertinent to the quantity of dietary carbohydrate required. In Gamble's studies with fasting subjects consuming 1200 cc of water daily, urinary water and electrolyte losses were minimized by the intake of salt and carbohydrate. Specifically, more body sodium and extracellular water were conserved through the intake of 100 gm glucose than by 4.5 gm of sodium chloride. When sodium chloride was given with glucose, all extracellular water loss was prevented. In subsequent studies of the effects of that level of dietary carbohydrate for minimum feeding concepts, Henschel et al.[53] ascertained that loss of speed and coordination experienced during fasting, and to some extent the ketosis, could be reversed by the daily administration of 100 g of sugar. In the meanwhile, field trials held in the tropics and arctic, where men were given only 60 gm of carbohydrate daily, showed that at that low level of intake, the calorie deficit and body weight loss were considerable and ketosis was not prevented systematically. Further laboratory studies showed that in young men receiving 250 gm of carbohydrate (1010 kg Cal) daily along with 4.5 gm of salt and a multivitamin supplement, no evidence of poor physiologic response to the stress of work was observed within twenty-four days.[54] At lower intakes of carbohydrate (580 kg Cal daily), pulmonary ventilation during work, pulse rate, and the oxygen debt showed a degree of deterioration during the first ten days. The authors concluded that when sufficient water, carbohydrate, salt, and vitamins are provided, ketosis, dehydration, and hypoglycemia are prevented under conditions of moderate energy expenditure, and performance capacity was well maintained up to a loss of 10 percent of initial body weight.

Establishing the minimum water requirements is relatively more difficult and complicated by the effects of work load and unanticipated environmental conditions which have a major impact on sweat rate and evaporative water loss. A preliminary study[55] was conducted with men consuming 1000 kg Cal daily of an all carbohydrate diet and drinking either 1800 cc or 900 cc of water daily. As compared with the intake of water *ad libitum*, the two reduced levels of water resulted in the conservation of body water through a reduction in insensible water loss at rest and sweat rate during work. Reduced rate of sweating resulted in a rise of body temperature during treadmill walking with increased pulse and respiration rates. However, performance on the treadmill was deemed to be adequate over a period of two to three weeks at the higher level of fluid intake. At the lower fluid intake there was a rapid rise in body temperature, particularly during work, which resulted in termination of the study within five days.

In a large number of cases, the addition of protein to low calorie diets has been attempted in order to avoid the excessive depletion of body protein. There is no significant difference in the urinary nitrogen excretion in subjects on a protein-free or protein-containing 900 kg Cal daily diet with either 1800 cc or 800 cc of water daily.[56, 57] But the diet containing meat protein was ketogenic and the increased solute load in the kidneys resulted in greater body water losses. A food energy intake of approximately 950 kg Cal daily appears to be the lowest level at which the addition of protein can produce a less negative nitrogen balance than an equivalent number of protein-free calories.[58] At that level of energy intake, a comparable reduction in the negativity of nitrogen balance is achieved with the inclusion of 3 or 6 gm of nitrogen in the diet, and small amounts of protein may be consumed without modification of urine volume.

Some consideration has also been given to the inclusion of some fat in low calorie diets for its protein-sparing effects; however, the consensus is that there is no important difference between fat or carbohydrate in that regard.[59]

Perhaps the greatest debate in minimal feeding concepts has centered upon the use of relatively high fat content, low calorie diets. Diets providing 1000 kg Cal daily and comprised of approximately 35 percent by weight of fat mixed with meat protein have been tested extensively.[60] That composition may be adequate for survival purposes for several weeks in relatively sedentary subjects, but in the author's personal experiences it augments the ketosis during the first two to five days of restricted feeding in combination with hard work and persistent nausea. In addition, for most people the mixture is not palatable when eaten cold. The inclusion of small amounts of fat to restricted diets, contributing some 10 to 20 percent of total calories, does not cause any undue physiologic compromise and seems to be a reasonable approach.

The effects of ketosis on physical performance and the considerable cost to body water and electrolytes in the urinary excretion of ketone bodies cannot be overemphasized. There appears to be some adaptation to increased rates of fat metabolism in that both blood level and urine output of ketones decrease during repeated fasts.[61, 62] Adrenalcortical hormones may inhibit ketosis;[63] anterior pituitary extracts produce ketonemia in fasting but not fed animals.[64] The ketogenic factor in meat protein has been partially isolated.[65] There are significant sex differences in the sensitivity to fasting ketosis; women suffer more from this reaction than do men[66] and excrete greater amounts of acetone in their urine.[67, 68, 69]

Overall, the intake of 1000 kg Cal daily (largely as carbohydrate) and 4.5 gm salt appears to be a minimum essential dietary for the maintenance of a good level of work performance capability in active men for a period of several weeks. Within this framework, the importance of all the vitamins has not been scientifically established, but parsimony would dictate the inclusion of a multivitamin tablet. Salt tablets are not well tolerated and enteric-coated pills tend to be excreted intact in the feces. However, beverages such as bouillons and soups are acceptable carriers for salt. Relatively low levels of fat in low calorie diets are well tolerated and may improve the palatability of the food. The significance of the addition of small amounts of protein to restricted diets is unclear. Up to 7 percent of calories from protein may be consumed without a substantive change in urine output. However, meat protein tends to be ketogenic, and therefore the use of casein has been suggested. It is important to bear in mind that the effects of protein insufficiency and negative nitrogen balance are delayed in terms of effects on fitness, and therefore beyond the realm of a practical short-term feeding concept.

Water requirements are largely a function of environmental conditions; the intake of 1800 cc daily appears to be adequate for nominal levels of work output for several weeks in a temperate environment; however, the requirement would increase dramatically with significantly elevated rates of water loss.

There are, of course, exceptional and heroic survival episodes which bring out the limits of human endurance. McGee[70] chronicled the case of a man, Pablo, lost in the desert of the southwestern U.S.A. at the turn of the century. When Pablo became lost he had only one day's supply of water with him, yet in the next eight days he rode thirty-five miles and walked or crawled 100 to 150 miles. He spent 170 hours without water with the exception of a few scorpions, insects, and his own urine which he drank for five days. On the eighth day he reached help, but by that time had lost thirty-five to forty pounds or approximately 25 percent of his initial body weight. He retained his "trail-sense" even though he was delirious. At that time it was generally considered that one-half the victims of "desert-thirst" would die within thirty-six hours, three-quarters within fifty hours, and all would be dead within eighty hours. Pablo, however, survived and regained his health. This particular case, although of considerable human interest, is of no value for planning a practical daily allotment of food or water. However, it points out the importance of a high level of motivation.

PERFORMANCE AND DIETARY SUPPLEMENTATION

A more vexing problem concerning nutrition and work performance has to do with less extreme conditions of malnutrition or conditions under which malnutrition is suspected but not proven. For those marginal nutritional states, could dietary supplementation lead to improved performance capacity? Within the same general context, do work performance and physical achievement impose special nutritional requirements in the relatively fit and apparently adequately nourished individual? A useful approach to the evaluation of this topic is to attempt to synthesize concepts which are both practical and scientifically defensible. Several theories which are offered for aiding work performance through supplementation with conventional foods are related to the renewal of supply of energy substrates and/or improvement or facilitation of biochemical pathways. Those theories, while oversimplified and on the surface naive, particularly in view of some of the time-dependent and nonlinear body responses, nevertheless provide a general framework for experimental testing. Research in this area requires rigorous standardization of testing procedures, and the avoidance of the influence of subject training effects and subjective impressions.

One important dietary consideration, then, is associated closely with the question of energy expenditure, calorie requirements, and the fuel for muscular exercise. In that regard, it is germane to review briefly the caloric requirements of a hypothetical, statistical construct, "the standard man," and arrive at some general approximations of his needs. If a person consumes a diet which conforms generally to the National Research Council's recommended dietary allowances, i.e. one which provides a nutrient intake for the maintenance of good nutrition in practically all healthy people in the U.S.A., what may be expected of his daily energy requirements? Tabled values compiled by the Food and Nutrition Board indicate a desirable intake of 2700 kg Cal daily for men between the ages of twenty-three and fifty years and 2000 kg Cal daily for women of a comparable age. Surely this reflects a low level of physical activity and the sedentary mode of life of most people. High levels of energy expenditure associated with active men and those engaged in heavy occupational work are reported to be in the range of 3400 to 3800 kg Cal/day. Those values are reasonably reliable since food intake data usually agrees with carefully taken time-motion studies of energy expenditure within 10 percent. Table V shows the breakdown of energy requirements for sedentary and active occupational groups, and it can be seen that the major differences are associated with the ex-

TABLE V

DAILY ENERGY REQUIREMENTS OF A CLERK AND A COAL MINER OF COMPARABLE AGE, HEIGHT, AND BODY WEIGHT[a]

Activity	Total Energy Requirements, kg Cal	
	Clerk	Coal Miner
1. Working	816	1700
2. In Bed; Daytime Dozing	544	527
3. Recreational and Off Work	1400	1556
TOTAL	2760	3783

[a]Garry, R. C., Passmore, R., Warnock, G. M., and Durnin, J. V. G. A.: *Med Res Council Spec Rep* 289. Her Majesty's Stat. Off. 1955.

penditure for daily work activities. For a detailed summary of the calorie cost of various activities, the interested reader is referred to an excellent review with some thirty-eight tables by Passmore and Durnin,[71] and an updating of the data by Buskirk.[72]

For a comparison of the physiologic cost of work performance, it is useful to relate rate of energy expenditure and the corresponding oxygen consumption to the individual's maximal oxygen uptake, e.g. the maximal aerobic work capacity. In this author's experience, male nonathletes aged twenty-eight to forty-five years who are brought into a good state of physical fitness through running and heavy calisthenics have an average maximum oxygen uptake of 3.4 l/min or approximately 42 to 45 cc O_2/kg body weight/min, as determined by treadmill testing. Those subjects can usually walk at rates and on grades eliciting a consumption of 50 percent of the maximal oxygen uptake for several hours daily with, of course, periodic rest periods (once an hour). For nominal body weights of 60 to 75 kg, that corresponds approximately to treadmill walking at 3.0 mph on an incline of 3 to 5°. The work would be largely aerobic and heart rate and body temperature would come into equilibrium in a new steady-state. The average energy cost of the activity is approximately 580 kg Cal/hr or 9 kg Cal/min, and it would be categorized by the subjects as moderate/heavy work. Treadmill walking at 2.6 to 3.0 mph at grades of 0 to 2° of incline elicits an oxygen consumption which is 32 percent of the maximal oxygen uptake; the average energy expenditure is 360 kg Cal/hr or 6 kg Cal/min and the activity is considered to be easy work. Many industrial workers, although not at the same high level of fitness as cited above, can expend energy at the rate of 5 to 6 kg Cal/min during daily work and sustain that level over many productive years. A significant departure may be found for those occupations requiring awkward positions or the repetitive use of certain muscle groups.

For the relatively low intensity and long duration work situation described above, which maximizes the daily calorie expenditure, the energy derived from protein metabolism provides an inconsequential fraction of the total requirements.

The original demonstration that nitrogen excretion is relatively unaffected by exercise is usually attributed to Pettenkofer and Voit.[73] Actually, there is a slight increase in the urinary nitrogen excretion for one to two days following heavy work, but the small rise is in no way related to the quantity of prior work performed. In exercising dogs[74] running continuously for ten hours or more at a work intensity which is 43 percent of the maximal oxygen uptake, protein metabolism contributes merely 3 to 4.5 percent of the gross energy requirement. Similar studies have been conducted with human volunteers; the cumulative urinary nitrogen excretion of resting and working human subjects is shown in Figure 2. Exercise consisted of easy treadmill walking with an average rate of expenditure of 360 kg Cal/hr; resting subjects were maintained in the near basal state with an average expenditure of 80 kg Cal/hr. The subjects were initially postabsorptive and were offered only water and salt for the period of the study. It can be seen in Figure 2 that nitrogen

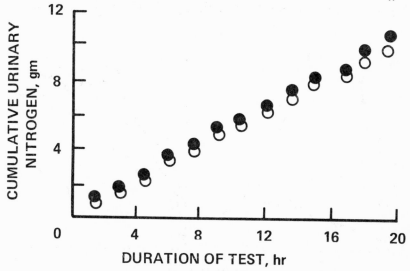

Figure 2. Cumulative urine nitrogen excretion in postabsorptive subjects. Urinary nitrogen in gm is shown on the vertical scale; test duration in hr is shown on the horizontal scale. Resting subjects are shown by open symbols; subjects walking on a treadmill are shown by closed symbols. (Young, D. R., et al. *J Appl Physiol, 21*:1047, 1966.)

output for the two levels of activity is substantially similar.

Body fats are oxidized extensively during work, largely in the form of circulating free fatty acids which are released from adipose tissue through lipolytic factors. Figure 3 shows the increase in serum levels of free fatty acids that may be expected in postabsorptive subjects as well as the influence of long duration easy treadmill walking. In resting subjects, the values rise to levels of 1.1 meq/l and then remain at the new steady-state level for several hours; in working subjects, the concentration reaches a level of 2.4 meq/l. Actually, for several minutes following the commencement of exercise, rate of lipolysis does not keep apace with fatty acid uptake and oxidation by muscle, and consequently there are transitory decreases in the plasma level of free fatty acids. However, beyond the initial period of adjustment, the level of free fatty acids rises and fat metabolism as determined by tracer kinetic studies tends to be maximized. Table VI shows the rate of body fat utilization which can be expected in the steady state with high levels of the plasma free

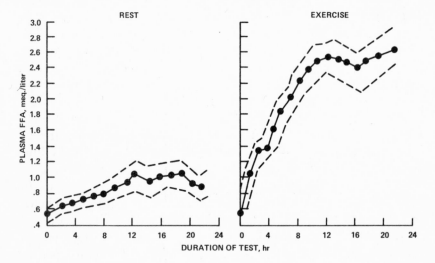

Figure 3. Plasma free fatty acids (FFA) in postabsorptive subjects. FFA in meq/liter is shown on the vertical scale; duration of test in hr is shown on the horizontal scale. The 95 percent confidence interval is shown. (Young, D. R., et al. *J Appl Physiol, 21*:1047, 1966.)

fatty acids and for work periods of up to thirteen hours duration. That data translates into some 22 to 25 g fat oxidized per hour by the muscles and represents 75 to 85 percent of total fat utilized. An additional 5 to 10 percent of lipid utilized is presumed to be derived directly from the fat stores within muscle; those fat depots are not in equilibrium with or at least do not exchange rapidly with the plasma free fatty acids. Studies by Havel et al.[75] for shorter periods of work show similar results. In that case, postabsorptive subjects walked for only two hours on a treadmill at an average rate of energy expenditure of 5 to 6 kg Cal/min; 41 to 49 percent of total CO_2 production was derived from the plasma free fatty acids. Those values approximate well the data obtained during longer duration work as shown in Table VI, and therefore the work period in itself is inconsequential in its effects on fatty acid oxidation over a two to thirteen hour time frame. Studies such as those cited above avoid excessive lactic acid accumulation and the inhibitory effect of lactate on lipolysis, and therefore maximize fat mobilization and oxidation. Significantly, there was no suggestion of a metabolic acidosis in the above studies.

In view of the preferential shift to fat metabolism during postabsorptive work, the use of high fat meals to augment performance has been tested by several investigators. Subjects maintained on high fat diets tend to consume slightly more oxygen during physical exercise than do subjects on a high carbohydrate diet.[76, 77] The differences are small, 8 to 11 percent, but consistent. Intakes of very high fat diets, providing in excess of 90 percent of calories as fat, decrease efficiency and work capacity during the course of a one and one half hour exercise test.[78] The loss of endurance is attributed in part to ketonemia. It can be shown that metabolic adjustments to ketonemia occur, particularly during starvation[79] wherein arteriovenous ketone differences of approximately 7 mg percent indicate a considerable uptake and utilization of ketone bodies by peripheral tissue. However, the significance of ketone body oxidation in the work day of the "standard man" is probably of no major consequence or importance. Most of the fat oxidized during work derives from the circulating free fatty acids; indeed, tracer studies cited in Table VI show that 75 percent of an

TABLE VI

TURNOVER RATE AND OXIDATION OF PLASMA FREE FATTY ACIDS (FFA) IN PHYSICALLY FIT SUBJECTS[a]

Level of Activity	No. of Subjects	Plasma FFA, meq/L	Fractional Rate of Disappearance of Plasma FFA, per Min	Fraction of Plasma FFA Oxidized, per Min	CO_2 Derived from FFA m Moles/Min	Total CO_2 Production m Moles/Min	CO_2 Derived from FFA %
Resting	2	2.4	0.246 - 0.263	0.073 - 0.091	3.98 - 5.00	10.7 - 13.2	37.2 - 37.8
Exercising	2	1.1	0.339 - 0.369	0.200 - 0.230	22.6 - 22.8	43.5 - 46.5	48.6 - 52.4

[a]Young, D. R., Shapira, J., Forrest, R., Adachi, R. R., Lim, R., and Pelligra, R.: *J Appl Physiol*, 23:716, 1967.

TABLE VII

TURNOVER RATE AND OXIDATION OF PLASMA GLUCOSE IN PHYSICALLY FIT SUBJECTS[a]

Level of Activity	No. of Subjects	Plasma Glucose	Fractional Rate of Disappearance of Plasma Glucose per Hr	Glucose Oxidation mg/Kg per Hr	CO_2 Derived from Glucose m Moles/Hr	Total CO_2 Production m Moles/Hr	CO_2 from Glucose, %
Resting	10	72 ± 5.6	0.411 ± 0.213	79.0 ± 28.3	204 ± 73	631 ± 72.0	33 ± 12.0
Exercising	10	69 ± 6.5	0.550 ± 0.154	175 ± 62.7	451 ± 152	2648 ± 249	17.0 ± 5.0

Values are means ± standard deviations.

[a]Young, D. R., Pelligra, R., Shapira, J., Adachi, R. R., and Skrettingland, K.: *J Appl Physiol, 23:*734, 1967.

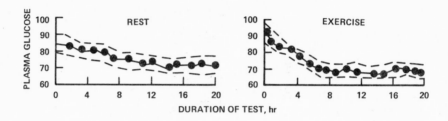

Figure 4. Plasma glucose in postabsorptive subjects. Glucose in mg/100 ml is shown on the vertical scale; duration of test in hr is shown on the horizontal scale. The 95 percent confidence interval is shown. (Young, D. R., et al. *J Appl Physiol, 21*:1047, 1966.)

intravenously administered test dose of uniformly labelled ^{14}C palmitate is eliminated ultimately as ^{14}C O_2.

Glucose oxidation proceeds at a fairly brisk rate during exercise. Figure 4 shows the general decline in the blood sugar level of postabsorptive subjects working at 32 percent of the maximal oxygen uptake. The level of glucose falls during the first nine to ten hours at a slightly faster rate than in resting subjects, and then reaches a new steady state level reflecting the balance between glucose utilization and production. The kinetic parameters for blood glucose utilization during prolonged work are shown in Table VII. As compared with resting subjects, the rate of glucose oxidation is doubled although only 17 percent of total CO_2 production arises from the blood sugar. That corresponds to a rate of glucose oxidation of 8 to 20 g/hr during work and it can be shown that 100 percent of an administered dose of uniformly labelled glucose can be expected to appear ultimately as ^{14}C O_2.

For easy to moderately heavy work of relatively short duration in the postabsorptive state, there is a simultaneous increased hepatic release of glucose[80, 81] as well as an increased uptake of glucose by the working muscles.[82] Occasional reports suggest that following several hours of work in the postabsorptive state, there is a glucose intolerance which persists for approximately one and one half days.[83]

During heavy work corresponding to 76 percent of the maximal oxygen uptake and representative of competitive cross-country skiing, muscle glycogen is depleted.[84] During the course of a 60 to 100 min work period on the bicycle ergometer, raising the work load from 28 percent to 54 percent of the maximal oxygen uptake increased the utilization of muscle glycogen from 0.31 to 0.83 g/100 g muscle/hr. When the work load was increased to 78 percent of the maximal oxygen uptake, muscle glycogen utilization rose to 1.56 g/100 g muscle. Following this heavy exercise and the relative depletion of muscle glycogen, the eating of high carbohydrate diets for several days leads to a greater deposition of glycogen in muscle than does the consumption of a mixed diet or one which is high in fat plus protein.[85] Furthermore, endurance was greater with a lesser decline in blood glucose following the high carbohydrate diet. In fact, exhaustive exercise time was in excess of 100 percent greater than in those subjects consuming either a mixed diet or a combination of fat plus protein. Thus supplemental dietary carbohydrate is of proven value for competitive sports.

For elevated rates of energy expenditure, the carbohydrate oxidized by muscle drives from two sources: (a) the blood glucose and (b) muscle glycogen via pathways related to glycogenolysis. The studies reported above show that the prefeeding of high carbohydrate diets under special circumstances has a decidedly beneficial effect on work performance. Over the range studied, the benefits of high carbohydrate meals probably have their greatest effects in very hard work situations and competitive sports. Supplementation of fit subjects with carbohydrate during easy treadmill walking raises the respiratory quotient towards unity indicating the trend towards carbohydrate oxidation. Havel et al.[86] provided 280 g of carbohydrate (1120 kg Cal) to test subjects during a five hour period of observation which included two hours of exercise. That quantity of carbohydrate, theoretically, should have supplied the total energy requirement. As a result, there was a striking decrease in the mobilization of free fatty acids so that less was available for oxidation by the working muscles. Under the conditions of the test, only 7 to 10 percent of CO_2 production arose from fatty acid oxidation. Underlying the above findings is the recurrent "carbohydrate theory" of fatigue. The studies which show a beneficial effect of carbohydrate diets have as their basis the degree and extent of blood glucose and muscle glycogen metabolism.

In another area, Haggard and Greenberg[87] reported a beneficial effect of between meal snacks on employee attitude and general performance in industrial work situations. However, the underlying causes of the reported improvements are not known. The psychomotor components (hand steadiness, short-term memory, reaction time) of fitness are remarkably stable in postabsorptive subjects during a nine hour period of work,[88] even though the blood sugar level declines steadily from 90 to 70 mg percent; therefore, the maintenance of blood sugar through frequency of feeding ordinarily would not be expected to have an influence in most people in light work situations. Decrements in psychomotor performance can be induced through the rapid IV administration of insulin and are first noted at blood sugar levels of 55 to 60 mg percent. These latter values are low, however, and are not expected to occur typically during the course of a working day. Relatively little is known about special dietary needs in industry; snacks between meals appear useful for industrial productivity but perhaps chiefly for psychological reasons.

Studies of relatively low intensity physical work do not point to any large benefits associated with recency of carbohydrate intake. In exercising dogs working at 43 percent of the maximal oxygen uptake, the provision of carbohydrate supplements during work does not materially increase the capacity for long duration exhaustive work,[89, 90] although with carbohydrate supplementation the decline of the blood sugar during work is not as extensive. The dogs were meal-eaters and consumed the daily balanced ration (~200 g) in a single meal. The effect of work performance in relationship to feeding time is shown in Table VIII. Work performed at four and six hours after eating is less efficient than work in the postabsorptive state or within one and one half hours following a large single meal, because oxygen consumption and energy expenditure for a fixed task were higher, heart rate was higher, and the rectal temperature rose to higher levels. Thus, this particular series showed no major improvements in objective work capacity

TABLE VIII

EFFECT OF PROXIMITY OF MEALTIME ON PHYSIOLOGIC
RESPONSES OF DOGS TO A 40-MINUTE TREADMILL TEST[a]

| | *Hours After Feeding* | | | |
	1 1/2	*4*	*6*	*24*
Mean Energy Expenditure, Kg Cal/Min	3.36	3.52	3.52	3.31
Respiratory Quotient	.93	.95	.91	.79
Pulse Rate/Min.	216	223	223	211
Δ Rectal Temp. °F	+0.9	+1.4	+1.6	+0.6

[a]Young, D. R. et al.: *J Appl Physiol, 14*:1013, 1959.

which could be attributed to dietary carbohydrate intake either in a meal or as a special food supplement.

Overall, the average person is apt to benefit marginally his work capacity through dietary modifications related to metabolic fuels and energy expenditure. Carbohydrates are the dietary components of choice. They minimize rate of decline of the blood glucose, spare muscle glycogen, and inhibit fat utilization. Light work loads will be performed relatively more efficiently, that is, at a lesser physiologic cost. For heavy work loads for the extremely fit subject, carbohydrate diets improve endurance capacity largely through their effect on blood glucose and muscle glycogen.

Exceptional cases are always noteworthy in that they may suggest unusual or unanticipated factors which shape or modify the relationships between diet and the state of physical fitness. The Masai tribe of Africa is a case in point. At the age of approximately fourteen years, boys are bound by tradition for the following two decades to consume a diet comprised almost exclusively of meat and dairy products. During that general period, time is spent tending cattle, seeking pasture, visiting friends, and seeking new relationships. For those activities, some twelve to twenty miles per day are covered at a brisk walk. The men are short in stature, 160 to 173 cm, lean, and attain body weights of only 130 to 140 pounds. The diet is strikingly different from that of a typical Western society. Protein intake (fatty meat and fermented whole milk) is high. In contrast to Western societies which obtain the major source of carbohydrates in the form of (a) vegetables, fruits, and from considerable quantities of the refined carbohydrates sucrose and starch in the form of soft drinks, confections, and desserts, and (b) foods based on cereals (bread, rice, noodles, spaghetti), the Masai consume largely lactose, the only major carbohydrate of animal origin. In the absence of a controlled and reproducible fermentation process, it is difficult to estimate the lactose or other carbohydrate content of the milk product consumed. Thirdly, the intake of relatively saturated fats and cholesterol is high although levels of blood lipids are low and therefore are in marked contrast to the findings of Ahrens et al.[91] who related low levels of the serum lipids to the consumption of polyunsaturated fats. With an abundant consumption of dairy products, up to 3 *l*/day of fermented whole milk, the intake of minerals would vary from high in calcium and phosphorus to marginal in other factors, according to prevailing Western opinion. Similarly, the intake of vitamin A would be adequate, but the consumption of other vitamins could be marginal. Again, these estimates are subject to considerable variations based upon the state of the products and quantities consumed and could only be determined with precision through controlled feeding studies and food analysis.

The population shows an exceptionally high state of physical fitness. In one particular series of tests,[92] the maximal oxygen consumption was determined utilizing the Balke[93] variation of treadmill testing. The maximal oxygen uptake specifically measures cardiorespiratory variables, but in a broader context it is taken as a measure of performance capacity. For population studies and screening purposes, the measurement of maximal oxygen uptake has the advantage of being relatively independent of skills, motivation, and emotionality. The Balke version of testing requires an increase in grade of 1%/min at a constant rate of walking, and provides the opportunity of assessing the time-history of the response as well as any transients of interest.

TABLE IX

RATING OF WORK CAPACITY WITH MAXIMAL OXYGEN UPTAKE

Max. O_2 Uptake, Cc/Kg/Min.	Balke Subjects Test Duration Min.	Rating of Work Capacity	Masai Subjects Test Duration Min.	Max. O_2 Uptake Cc/Kg/Min.
≤ - 25	≤ - 8	Inferior		
25 - 30	8 - 11	Very Poor		
30 - 35	12 - 14	Poor		
35 - 40	15 - 17	Fair		
40 - 45	18 - 20	Good	24	40 (> 44)
45 - 50	21 - 23	Very Good		
50 - 55	24 - 26	Excellent	36	55 (14 - 19)
55 +	27 +	Superior	39	59 (20 - 43)

Age of Masai subjects is shown in parentheses.

A group of fifty-three Masai men, fourteen to sixty-four years of age, was studied. Table IX compares the work capacity and fitness scores developed by Balke in studies with 530 male subjects with those measured in the Masai. For Masai men between the ages of fourteen and forty-three years, the maximal oxygen uptake was relatively constant, 55 to 59 cc O_2/min/kg body weight. Beyond the age of forty-four years, the uptake was 40 cc O_2/kg body weight. Values of 55 to 59 cc O_2/kg are remarkably high and indeed are in the range shown by Olympic class athletes. Not only are the oxygen uptakes relatively high, but endurance time is considerable, indicating the capacity to sustain and endure oxygen debt and lactic acid accumulation as the limit of aerobic capacity is reached. By those criteria these subjects would be judged to be exceptionally fit.

Since pulmonary ventilation and diffusion are not likely to be limiting factors in the exercise capacity of those subjects, the high level of performance must involve primarily the circulation. Clinical evaluations[94] in 386 subjects showed no evidence of the development of hypertension with increasing age or increases in level of serum cholesterol. In fact, the blood cholesterol is low in subjects aged fourteen to fifty-five or more years, seldom attaining levels higher than 150 mg percent, and there is remarkably little heart disease as assessed from the electrocardiogram. The hearts and aortae of fifty Masai men were collected at autopsy.[95] The aorta showed extensive lipid infiltration and fibrous changes, but very few complicated lesions that would give rise to thrombosis. The coronary arteries showed intimal thickening which equaled that of older U.S. men; however, between the ages of twenty and sixty years, the Masai vessels *enlarge* and therefore provide a greater flow capacity to the myocardium.

Thus, two of the circulatory parameters which may be associated with the considerable work capacity are the stable and relatively low blood pressures throughout most of the life which provide a considerable cardiovascular reserve, and enlargement of the coronary vessels with improved perfusion of the heart. It is not clear how the state of physical fitness is achieved or maintained in these subjects nor the extent that genetic factors, nutrition, or other environmental conditions influence their responses.

One final dietary supplement deserves mention because of the substantial research efforts directed towards the demonstration of a positive effect on work performance. Phosphate beverages are considered by many to be exhilirating. In approximately 1916, studies were initiated in Germany with large numbers of volunteers to evaluate the effect of phosphates on muscular performance. The underlying theory was as follows: Since muscle depends upon phosphorylation reactions to provide energy for contractility and the performance of physical work, increasing the dietary supply of soluble phosphates could theoretically increase performance. Early laboratory and field trials of the effect of acid sodium phosphate (NaH_2PO_4) supplements showed promising results. The literature as reviewed by Keys[96] shows a subsequent wide acceptance by athletes and for all types of fatigue and debility. Although the findings have not been systematic, and in view of the relative lack of well-documented studies showing a consistent beneficial effect of phosphates on objective work capacity and the likely mechanisms of action, there is a general skepticism of any effect of a high phosphorus intake on muscular performance. On the one hand, the likelihood of phosphorus deficiencies in adults on ordinary diets should be remote; secondly, the possibility of increasing the phosphorus content in muscle of people eating normal dietaries is indeed slim; therefore, there is probably little chance of promoting performance through facilitating the formation of organic phosphates in tissue simply by an abundant intake of the water soluble phosphates.

During the past several years, man's curiosity has drawn him into new and unusual environments. Exploration of the moon and the weightless environment of space elicited a series of physiologic responses which suggested the need for dietary modification. Experiences during space flight demonstrated bone mineral losses, weakness in special muscle groups (extensors in the arms and legs), losses of red blood cell mass, cardiovascular deconditioning, and electrolyte losses. The losses of potassium as reviewed by Berry and Smith[97] are a case in point. At least two factors give rise to body potassium loss. On the one hand, some muscle disuse-type atrophy contributes to the loss. Secondly, one of the early responses to the state of zero gravity is thought to be a redistribution of the circulating blood volume from the lower extremities to the chest and neck regions with a resulting increased right atrial filling, a decrease in the pituitary secretion of antidiuretic hormone, and a decrease in aldosterone production. The net result is an increased loss of water, sodium, and potassium through the kidneys. The kidney has apparently little capacity to reabsorb and conserve potassium so that potassium losses continue unabated. A postulated effect of potassium loss and hypokalemia is to increase the irritability of the heart with a tendency towards disorders of cardiac rhythm. Indeed, certain cardiac arrhythmias were noted in the Apollo XV astronauts. During the eleven day Apollo XVI mission, the requirement was established for 140 meq of potassium daily during flight and 145 to 155 meq daily during the time spent on the lunar surface. In order to achieve the desired intake, several beverages were fortified with potassium gluconate. Assessment of the efficacy of the dietary regimen was based upon postflight measurements of the body exchangeable potassium pool. Measurements of total body potassium by K^{42} dilution studies revealed no loss in body potassium, and that was attributable directly to the increased dietary intake. This special problem focuses attention on the influence of electrolytes on performance capabilities, and the extent to which dietary intervention may significantly offset environmentally induced changes.

REFERENCES

1. Young, D. R. and Spector, H.: Physical performance capacity and nutriture: Evaluation of rations by animal experimentation. *Am J Nutrition, 5*:129-140, 1957.
2. Préobrajensky, B. S. and Baranova, L. T.: Des alterations anatomopathologiques de l'appareil audifit dans le jeunne aigu, d'apres des expériences animales portant sur le cobaye et a la souris blanche. *Acta Otolaryngol* (Stockh), *18*:1-20, 1932.
3. Cameron, A. T. and Carmichael, J.: The effect of acute starvation on the body organs of the adult white rat, with special reference to the adrenal glands. *Can J Res, 24*:37-48, 1946.
4. Morgulis, S.: *Fasting and Undernutrition.* New York, Dutton, 1923.
5. Krieger, M.: Ueber die atrophie des menschlichen organe bei inanition. *Arch Angew Anat, 7*:87-134, 1921.
6. Kerpel-Fronius, E.: Infantile mortality in Budapest in the year 1945 as reflected by the material of the children's clinic of the University. *J Pediatr, 30*:244-249, 1947.
7. Robins, G. N.: The fasting man. *Br Med J, 1*:1440-1446, 1890.
8. Benedict, F. G.: A study of prolonged fasting. Washington, Carnegie Inst., Pub. No. 280, 1915, 416 pp.
9. Keys, A., Brôzek, J., Henschel, A., Mickelson, O., and Taylor, H. L.: *The Biology of Human Starvation*, volume 1. Minneapolis, U of Minn Pr, 1950.
10. Benedict: Prolonged fasting.
11. Keys et al.: *Bio. Human Starvation.*
12. Addis, T., Poo, L. J., and Lew, W.: The quantities of protein lost by the various organs and tissues of the body during a fast. *J Biol Chem, 115*:111-116, 1936.
13. Addis, T., Poo, L. J., and Lew, W.: Protein loss from liver during a two-day fast. *J Biol Chem, 115*:117-121, 1936.
14. Taylor, H. L., Henschel, A., Mickelson, O., and Keys, A.: Some effects of acute starvation with hard work on body weight, body fluids, and metabolism. *J Appl Physiol, 6*:613-623, 1954.
15. White A.: Integration of the effects of adrenal cortical, thyroid and growth

hormones in fasting metabolism. *Recent Prog Hormone Res, IV*:153-181, 1949.

16. Meites, J. and Wolterink, L. F.: Uptake of radioactive iodine by the thyroids of underfed rats. *Science, 111*:175-176, 1950.

17. Meites, J. and Agrawala, I. P.: Effects of underfeeding on thiouracil action in rats and mice. *Endocrinology, 45*:148-152, 1949.

18. Cameron and Carmichael: Effect of acute starvation.

19. Handler, P. and Georgiade, R. S.: Influence of previous dietary protein and of ACTH on blood glucose concentration of fasting rats. *Am J Physiol, 164*:131-136, 1951.

20. Mulinos, M. G. and Pomerantz, L.: Pseudo-hypophysectomy, a condition resembling hypophysectomy produced by malnutrition. *J Nutrition, 19*:493-504, 1940.

21. D'Angleo, S. A., Gordon, A. S., and Charipper, H. A.: The effect of inanition on the anterior pituitary-adrenocortical interrelationship in the guinea pig. *Endocrinology, 42-43*:399-411, 1948.

22. MacLeod, J. J. R. and Prendergast, D. G.: Glycogen in the heart and skeletal muscles in starved and well-fed animals. *Proc R Soc Can, 15*:37-40, 1921.

23. Adrouny, G. A. and Russell, J. A.: Growth hormone and myocardial glycogen. *Fed Proc, 13*:1, 1954.

24. Werner, S. C.: Failure of gonadotrophic function of the rat hypophysis during chronic inanition. *Proc Soc Exp Biol Med, 41*:101-105, 1939.

25. Maddock, W. O. and Heller, C. G.: Dichotomy between hypophyseal content and amount of circulating gonadotrophins during starvation. *Proc Soc Exp Biol Med, 66*:595-598, 1947.

26. Eeg-Olofsson, R.: Plasma-proteins in epileptics during inanition. *Acta Med Scand, 106*:254-260, 1941.

27. Sunderman, F. W.: Studies in serum electrolytes. XIV: Changes in blood and body fluids in prolonged fasting. *Am J Clin Path, 17*:169-180, 1947.

28. Van Slyke, D. D. and Meyer, S. M.: The effects of feeding and fasting on the amino acid content of the tissues. *J Biol Chem, 16*:231-233, 1913-14.

29. Lennox, W. G., O'Connor, M., and Bellinger, M.: Chemical changes in the blood during fasting in the human subject. *Arch Intern Med, 38*:553-565, 1926.

30. Lennox, W. G.: Increase of the uric acid in the blood during prolonged starvation. *JAMA, 82*:602-604, 1924.

31. Lennox, W. G.: A study of the retention of uric acid during fasting. *J Biol Chem, 66*:521-572, 1925.

32. Eisenstein, A. B.: Current concepts of gluconeogenesis. *Am J Clin Nutr, 20*:282-289, 1967.

33. Feliz, P., Marliss, E., Owen, O. E., and Cahill, G. F.: Blood glucose and gluconeogenesis in fasting man. *Arch Intern Med, 123*:293-298, 1969.

34. Seubert, W. and Huth, W.: On the mechanism of gluconeogenesis and its

46   *Physical Performance, Fitness, and Diet*

regulation. *Biochem Z, 343*:176-191, 1965.
35. Dible, J. H.: Fat mobilization in starvation. *J Path Bact, 35*:451-466, 1932.
36. Pfeiffer, L.: Ueber den fettenbehalt des karpers und verschiedener Theile desselben bei mageren und fetten thieren. *Z Biol, 5*:340-380, 1887.
37. Keys et al.: *Bio. Human Starvation.*
38. Mendel, L. B. and Rose, W. C.: Inanition and the creatine content of muscle. *J Biol Chem, 10*:255-264, 1911.
39. Beattie, J., Herbert, P. H., and Bell, D. J.: Famine oedema. *Br J Nutrition, 2*:47-65, 1948.
40. McCance, R. A. and Widdowson, E. M.: Body compartments. *Proc R Soc Lond, 138*:115-130, 1951.
41. Keys et al.: *Bio. Human Starvation.*
42. Beattie et al.: Famine oedema.
43. Jensen, P.: Ueber den glycogenstaffwechsel des herzens. *Hoppe-Selye Zeit Gesamt Physiol, 35*:514-524, 1902.
44. Sunderman: Studies in serum electrolytes.
45. Keys et al.: *Bio. Human Starvation.*
46. Walters, J. H., Rossiter, R. J., and Lehmann, H.: Malnutrition in Indian prisoners of war in the Far East. *Lancet, 1*:205-210, 1947.
47. Bruckner, W. J., Wies, C. H., and Lavietes, P. H.: Anorexia nervosa and pituitary cachexia. *Am J Med Sci, 196*:663-673, 1938.
48. LeBlanc, J., Stewart, M., Marier, G., and Whillans, M. G.: Studies on acclimatization and on the effect of ascorbic acid in men exposed to cold. *Can J Biochem Physiol, 32*:407-427, 1954.
49. Taylor, et al.: Some effects of acute starvation.
50. Taylor, H. L., Brôzek, J., Henschel, A., Mickelsen, O., and Keys, A.: Effects of successive fasts on ability of men to withstand fasting during hard work. *Am J Physiol, 143*:148-155, 1945.
51. Guetzkow, H., Taylor, H. L., Brôzek, J., and Keys, A.: Relationship of speed of motor reaction to blood sugar level during acute starvation in man. *Fed Proc, 4*:28, 1945.
52. Gamble, J. L.: Physiologic information from studies on the life raft ration. *The Harvey Lecture Series, 42*:247-273, 1946-47.
53. Henschel, A., Taylor, H. L., and Keys, A.: Performance capacity in acute starvation with hard work. *J Appl Physiol, 6*:624-633, 1954.
54. Taylor, H. L., Buskirk, E. R., Brôzek, J., Anderson, J. T., and Grande, F.: Performance capacity and effects of caloric restriction with hard physical work on young men. *J Appl Physiol, 10*:421-429, 1957.
55. Grande, F., Taylor, H. L., Anderson, J. T., Buskirk, E., and Keys, A.: Water exchange in men on restricted water intake and a low calorie carbohydrate diet accompanied by physical work. *J Appl Physiol, 12*:202-210, 1958.
56. Quinn, M., Kleeman, C. R., Bass, D. E., and Henschel, A.: Nitrogen, water and electrolyte metabolism on protein and protein-free low-calorie diets in man; water restriction. *Metabolism, 3*:49-67, 1954.

57. Quinn, M., Kleeman, C. R., Bass, D. E., and Henschel, A.: Nitrogen, water and electrolyte metabolism on protein and protein-free low-calorie diets in man; adequate water intake. *Metabolism, 3*:68-77, 1954.
58. Calloway, D. H. and Spector, H.: Nitrogen balance as related to caloric and protein intake in active young men. *Am J Clin Nutrition, 2*:405-411, 1954.
59. Munro, H. N.: Carbohydrate and fat as factors in protein utilization and metabolism. *Physiol Rev, 31*: 449-488, 1951.
60. Drury, H. F., Vaughan, D. A., and Hannon, J. P.: Some metabolic effects of a high-fat, high-protein diet during semistarvation under winter field conditions. *J Nutrition, 67*:85-97, 1959.
61. Taylor, et al.: Effects of successive fasts.
62. Folin, O. and Denis, W.: On starvation and obesity with special reference to acidosis. *J Biol Chem, 21*:183-192, 1915.
63. Scott, J. L., Jr. and Engel, F. L.: The influence of the adrenal cortex and cold stress on fasting ketosis in the rat. *Endocrinol, 53*:410-422, 1953.
64. Bahner, F. W. R. and Taylor, N. R. W.: Fasting ketosis in hypophysectomized and normal rats. *Q J Exp Physiol, 37*:221-223, 1952.
65. Stewart, H. B. and Young, F. G.: A substance in animal tissues which stimulates ketone-body excretion. *Nature, 170*:976-978, 1952.
66. Deuel, H. J., Jr. and Gulick, M.: Studies on ketosis. I. The sexual variation in starvation ketosis. *J Biol Chem, 96*:25-34, 1932.
57. Mackay, E. M. and Sherill, J. W.: A comparison of the ketosis developed during fasting by obese patients and normal subjects. *Endocrinology, 21*:677-680, 1937.
68. Heinbecker, P.: Studies on metabolism of Eskimos. *J Biol Chem, 80*:461-475, 1928.
69. Hawley, E. E., Johnson, C. W., and Murlin, J. R.: The possibility of glyconeogenesis from fat. II. The effect of high fat diets on the respiratory metabolism and ketosis of man. *J Nutrition, 6*:523-557, 1933.
70. McGee, W. J.: Desert thirst as disease. *Interst Med J, 13*:279-300, 1906.
71. Passmore, R. and Durnin, J. V. G. A.: Human energy expenditure. *Physiol Rev, 35*:801-840, 1955.
72. Buskirk, E. R.: Problems related to the caloric cost of living. *Bull N Y Acad Med, 36*:365-388, 1960.
73. Pettenkofer, M. and Voit, C.: Untersuchungen uber den Stoffverbrauch des Normalen Menschen. *Z Biol, 2*:537-543, 1866.
74. Young, D. R. and Price, R.: Utilization of body energy reserves during work in dogs. *J Appl Physiol, 16*:351-354, 1961.
75. Havel, R. J., Naimark, A., and Borchgrevink, C. F.: Turnover rate and oxidation of free fatty acids of blood plasma in man during exercise: Studies during continuous infusion of palmitate-1-C^{14}. *J Clin Invest, 42*:1054-1063, 1963.

76. Krogh, A. and Lindhard, J.: The relative value of fat and carbohydrate as sources of muscular energy. *Biochem J, 14*:290-296, 1920.
77. Bierring, E.: The respiratory quotient and the efficiency of moderate exercise measured in the initial state and in the steady state during postabsorptive conditions. *Arbeitsphysiology, 5*:17-24, 1932.
78. Christensen, E. H. and Hansen, O.: III. Arbeitsfahigkeit und Ernahrung. *Scand Arch Physiol, 81*:160-171, 1939.
79. Gammeltoft, A.: The significance of ketone bodies in fat metabolism. *Acta Physiol Scand, 19*:270-279, 1950.
80. Reichard, G. A., Issekutz, B., Jr., Kimbel, P., Putnam, R. C., Hochella, N. J., and Weinhouse, S.: Blood glucose metabolism in man during muscular work. *J Appl Physiol, 16*:1001-1005, 1961.
81. Wahren, J., Ahlborg, G., Felig, P., and Jorfeldt, L.: Glucose metabolism during exercise in man. *Adv Exp Med Biol, 11*:189-203, 1971.
82. Sanders, C. A., Levinson, G. E., Abelmann, W. H., and Freinkel, N.: Effect of exercise on the peripheral utilization of glucose in man. *N Engl J Med, 271*:220-225, 1964.
83. Courtice, F. C. and Douglas, C. G.: The effects of prolonged muscular exercise on the metabolism. *Proc R Soc Lond (Biol), 119*:381-439, 1936.
84. Hermansen, L., Hultman, E., and Saltin, B.: Muscle glycogen during prolonged severe exercise. *Acta Physiol Scand, 71*:129-139, 1967.
85. Bergstrom, J., Hermansen, L., Hultman, E., and Saltin, E.: Diet, muscle glycogen and physical performance. *Acta Physiol Scand, 71*:140-150, 1967.
86. Havel, Naimark, and Borchgrevink: Turnover rate and oxidation.
87. Haggard, H. L. and Greenberg, L. A.: Between-meal feeding in industry: Effects on absenteeism and attitude of clerical employees. *J Am Diet Assoc, 15*:435-438, 1939.
88. Coler, C. R., McLaurin, W. A., and Young, D. R.: Effects of adrenalin or insulin on the performance of working and resting subjects. *Aerospace Med, 36*:1181-1186, 1965.
89. Young, D. R., Iacovino, A., Erve, P., Mosher, R., and Spector, H.: Effect of time after feeding and carbohydrate or water supplement on work in dogs. *J Appl Physiol, 14*:1013-1017, 1959.
90. Young, D. R., Schafer, N. S., and Price, R.: Effect of nutrient supplements during work on performance capacity in dogs. *J Appl Physiol, 15*:1022-1026, 1960.
91. Ahrens, E. H., Hirsch, J., Insull, W., Tsaltas, T. T., Blomstrand, R., and Peterson, M. L.: The influence of dietary fats on serum-lipid levels in man. *Lancet, 1*, Issue No. 6976:943-953, 1957.
92. Mann, G. V., Shaffer, R. D., and Rich, A.: Physical fitness and immunity to heart-disease in *Masai. Lancet, 2*, Issue No. 7426:1308-1310, 1965.
93. Balke, B. and Ware, R. W.: An experimental study of "physical fitness" of Air Force personnel. *U S Armed Forces Med J, 10*:675-688, 1959.
94. Mann, G. V., Shaffer, R. D., Anderson, R. S., and Sanstead, H. H.:

Cardiovascular disease in the *Masai. J Atheroscler Res, 4*:289-312, 1964.
95. Mann, G. V., Spoerry, A., Gray, M., and Jarashow, D.: Atherosclerosis in the *Masai. Am J Epidemiol, 95*:26-37, 1972.
96. Keys, A.: Physical performance in relationship to diet. *Fed Proc, 2*:164-187, 1943.
97. Berry, C. A. and Smith, M.: What we've learnt from space exploration. *Nutrition Today,* 4-32, Sept./Oct. 1972.

Chapter 3

PERFORMANCE AND
BODY COMPOSITION

OVERWEIGHT and frank obesity have been the subjects of considerable research efforts since the 1950's. With regard to the influence on performance, the two aspects of weight gain which have been investigated are (a) the effect of body composition, that is, fat content, as well as (b) the effect of the burden of additional weight. The physiologic responses to treadmill exercise are related characteristically to the gross body weight. Therefore, at fixed grades and speeds, heavier subjects show a greater pulmonary ventilation, oxygen consumption, and an elevated pulse rate as compared to lighter weight personnel. Figure 5 shows the energy expenditure of one subject at first with and then without a 20 pound pack carried high across the shoulders. The speed of progression was varied from a very slow to a fast walk. The relationship between energy expenditure and speed of walking is generally curvilinear with a disproportionately high energy cost at the higher speeds. Thus one general effect of overweight is an increase in the physiologic cost of those activities related to locomotion. Bloom and Eidex[1] pointed out a similar set of responses in comparing energy expenditure in the obese and lean. However, their data showed that the obese individual tolerates his weight and responds better than a lean person carrying a load to provide a total weight equal to that of the obese. But the use of added loads to evaluate physiologic responses to exercise is not uncomplicated. For example, loads about the hips elicit a greater energy expenditure than comparable weights borne across the shoulders. That may be related to the effect of modification of the center of mass of the body. That factor, in addition to the curvilinear relationship between activity level and energy cost, cautions us that the conventional "pack test" for lean or normal weight subjects may be inappropriate in its application

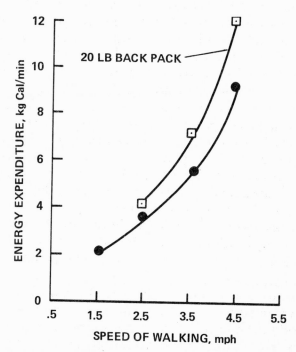

Figure 5. Effect of load carrying on energy expenditure during treadmill walking on a horizontal surface in a twenty-three-year-old man. Energy expenditure in kg Cal/min is shown on the vertical scale; speed of walking in mph is shown on the horizontal scale.

to studies of the effect of weight gain.

Even in relatively static physical work situations, the energy cost to the obese individual is higher. Åstrand et al.[2] studied the oxygen intake of obese men and women when working at constant submaximal loads of 300 kpm/min on the bicycle ergometer. In general, the responses were some 13 to 18 percent higher than their control counterparts.

Interpretation of the studies cited above is complicated by the relative lack of physical fitness in most obese subjects and therefore the expected loss of physiologic economy. Buskirk and Taylor[3] conducted one of the earlier studies which separated the variables of fitness and body composition. The maximal oxygen uptake was measured during treadmill tests in fifteen fit subjects who were participants in organized collegiate sports. They were twenty-two years of age, average height was 177.1 cm, body weight was 75.8 kg, and they bore 7.8 percent of body weight as fat. The thirty-nine sedentary subjects were similar in all dimensions with the exception of body fat content which averaged 15.9 percent of body weight. The maximal oxygen uptake of the fit group was 52.8 cc O_2/kg/min and was higher than the average value of 44.0 cc O_2/kg/min measured in the sedentary test group. The relatively inactive population was evaluated independently, and divided into subgroups with <10 percent fat, 10 to 25 percent fat, and >25 percent body fat content. The maximal oxygen uptake, on a fat-free body weight basis, was substantially similar (51 to 52 cc/kg/min) in the three groups. Therefore, it was concluded that the presence of excess fat per se does not have an important influence on the capacity of the cardiovascular-respiratory system to deliver oxygen to the working muscles under maximal performance conditions.

Another approach to the evaluation of the influence of body fat content on performance was undertaken with experimental adult dogs studied during treadmill running. The level of physical fitness was maintained constant through daily sessions of running,[4] and during a three-month experimental period of weight gain, the daily allotment of food was increased every ten days by an additional 50 gm/day until the body weights stabilized at a higher level. The submaximal work load (43% of maximal oxygen uptake) was held constant by adjusting the degree of incline for differences in body weight in order to achieve a constant work load of 202.9 kg-m/min. In this particular species, the relationship between work load and energy cost is clearly linear,[5] and consequently not complicated by those factors which lead to inordinate energy costs in man. The responses of the test dogs are shown in Table X. Despite the approximate 20 percent increase in body weight, oxygen consumption and heart rate remained relatively constant for fixed work loads.

Thus, in the overall, the overweight subject is under a substantial handicap in performance associated with locomotion because of a general lack of physical fitness and because of the

TABLE X

BODY WEIGHT GAIN AND PHYSIOLOGIC RESPONSES TO
A 50-MINUTE TREADMILL TEST (202.9 KG-M/MIN) IN
EIGHT BEAGLE DOGS

Body Wt., kg	10.36	12.40
O_2 Uptake, cc/min	748	753
Work Pulse Rate/min	225	230
Recovery Pulse Rate/min*	167	174

*Mean 4-min recovery pulse

additional burden of weight. Variation of body fat content from
10 to 25$^+$ percent does not in itself interfere with maximal or
submaximal cardiorespiratory performance. However, it is clear
that at some point in frank obesity there will be an altered
tolerance for work, possibly through loss of vital capacity from
encroachment by omental and mediastinal fat on the thoracic
space.

Total food deprivation has been recommended as a treatment
for frank obesity. Figure 6 shows the results of some of the
recent trials in that regard. Although more extensive data are
required in order to establish precise relationships regarding
rate of body weight loss during fasting, the results suggest that
in subjects confined to metabolic ward conditions, the rate of
weight loss in obese patients may be only somewhat less than
that expected in normal weight subjects.

Physical exercise during food restriction promotes the loss of
body weight, but not to the extent anticipated. Carlson and
Fröberg[6] studied twelve healthy men who walked 50 km/day
for ten days without food. The loss in ten days was 9.6 percent
of initial body weight which is similar to the loss shown in
sedentary subjects (Figure 6). In normal weight fasting dogs[7]
studied over a five-day period, body weight loss was 10 percent
under conditions of low daily levels of energy expenditure and
12.7 percent with high daily levels of energy expenditure. In
obese subjects maintained on restricted calorie diets, weight loss
and especially fat loss tended to be greater during the treatment

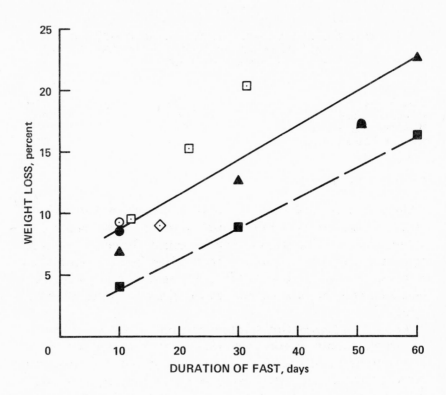

Figure 6. Percent body weight loss during fasting in sedentary subjects. Percent weight loss is shown on the vertical scale; duration of fast in days is shown on the horizontal scale.

period which included a seven and one half mile walk daily,[8] and exercise contributed more to body weight loss when caloric intake was restricted moderately than when restriction was more severe, <1000 kg Cal/day.

Exception has been taken with the probable clinical value of prolonged fasting for weight reduction because of the accompanying losses of lean body mass. Nitrogen loss during starvation in the obese subject is not particularly different during either sedentary or exercising[9] conditions nor from that observed in normal weight individuals. Body potassium loss during fasting is also substantially similar in obese and normal weight subjects.[10, 11] It would be desirable to minimize the extent of nonfat tissue loss which is expected to occur during long-term treatments by dietary reduction and special feeding schedules. The weight loss in obese subjects maintained on a mixed diet providing 800 kg calorie, 8 gm nitrogen daily,[12] can be divided into two phases: A period of rapid weight loss lasting three to six days and due principally to water loss, followed by an approximately constant rate of loss for several months in which primarily fat is lost with a variable loss of water and lean tissue. Birkenhager et al.[13] studied the effects of alternating periods of starvation and restricted feeding (680 kg Cal daily) of a mixed diet in obese subjects. The loss of fat accounted for 60 to 80 percent of the reduction in gross body weight over the period of observation; the negative nitrogen balance induced by intermittent starvation was not influenced by different levels of protein intake during the intervals between fasting. However, dietary supplementation with potassium during starvation minimized the absolute loss of potassium. In another study of intermittent starvation with obese subjects,[14] the effect of sixteen days of starvation preceded or followed by a two-week period of calorie restriction (600 to 800 kg Cal daily) was evaluated. The marked loss of weight and lean tissue occurring during starvation was of the same magnitude whether or not starvation was initiated after *ad libitum* feeding or after caloric restriction. However, during two weeks of initial calorie restriction, 70 percent of weight loss was adipose tissue, whereas during sixteen days of total starvation less than 15 percent of the lost tissue was fat. During poststarvation calorie restriction there was a reaccumulation of lean tissue but a loss of fat at a rate substantially greater than that observed during fasting.

Ketogenic restricted calorie diets would be useful for promoting weight loss because of their influence in modifying body compositional changes. For example, again for short periods of time (ten days), the loss of total body potassium while fasting was 15.1 gm in contrast to no loss during a period of intake of 1000 kg Cal daily of a high fat diet.[15] Furthermore, the body fat losses were greater during the high fat ketogenic period with only negligible changes in lean body mass, as compared with the results obtained on a 1000 kg Cal/day mixed diet.

Problems are encountered with obese subjects in arriving at reliable estimates of the degree of calorie imbalance, more precisely, the energetics associated with weight reduction regimens.[16] The materials balance technique would be a useful approach to attempt to explain the greater weight losses measured during moderate calorie restriction than during starvation, as well as the enhancement of fat loss by ketogenic diets. However, as pointed out by Buskirk and colleagues,[17] the ability to establish with precision the trends of calorie expenditure as well as the exact relationship between extent of weight loss, changes in body composition (water, fat, lean body weight), and its caloric equivalent may be lost in the "noise level" of the accuracy and reliability of the methodologies. Thus, because of associated measurement errors, balance studies sometimes present untenable results which defy thermodynamic principles; these are related to the lack of precision and accuracy in the measurement techniques.

In view of the probably chronic nature of the treatment of obesity through restricted feeding, exercise in combination with calorie restriction would be a useful adjunct for promoting weight loss.[18] In a limited number of cases, it has been shown to be effective in subjects maintained on 1000 to 1500 kg Cal daily of a mixed diet. For long-term studies, the problems of adequate mineral nutrition could become severe and special dietary supplements would be required. The use of high fat, low calorie diets in conjunction with moderate to hard work is debatable in view of the expected metabolic acidosis and malaise.

Exercise such as walking in obese subjects is of course not without its problems and complications. Chafing and foot blisters are encountered frequently as well as difficulties in maintaining body balance and stability during treadmill walking. Therefore, patience and discipline are further requirements for successful treatment through a planned exercise program.

Body fat loss during food deprivation in conjunction with exercise is a significant fraction of the weight loss in the obese, and a number of studies have been undertaken to evaluate fatty acid mobilization and utilization. At first, Gordon[19] demonstrated that obese subjects have higher postabsorptive plasma levels of free fatty acids than do nonobese people, but the plasma levels showed no systematic increase during a standard period of fasting. Also, the blood level of ketones changed slightly, if at all, during a one-week period of maintenance on a 1000 kg Cal/day high fat diet; in contrast, in the nonobese, the blood level of ketone bodies rises. Nineteen percent of obese subjects tested failed to show the expected rise in level of plasma fatty acids following the administration of epinephrine.[20] The data were taken as a partial explanation for the brittle or resistant weight loss shown by some obese subjects. The rate of conversion of labelled palmitate to CO_2 was at first shown to be lower in obese subjects,[20] but subsequent studies showed no important differences.[21, 22] In a more comprehensive evaluation of fatty acid metabolism, the oxidation rate of free fatty acids was shown to be 0.27 meq/min in five lean subjects and 0.27 meq/min in four obese subjects tested.[23] Thus the more recent evidence shows that rate of dissipation of fat through oxidative processes is substantially similar in obese and normal subjects under general resting conditions.

Effect of exercise in combination with restricted food intake on fatty acid mobilization in the obese has also been evaluated.[24] Following a total of four hours of exercise on the treadmill and bicycle ergometer, the plasma level of free fatty acids was in the range of 1.74 to 1.82 meq/l, and substantially similar to measured values in normal weight subjects. However, the resting level of free fatty acids increased sequentially in obese subjects during partial food restriction (600 to 800 kg Cal/day) as well as during total food deprivation, and therefore the differences between pre- and postexercise values were smaller than expected normally. When the obese patients entered the recovery phase of testing with an approximately normal caloric intake, the resting level of free fatty acids was reduced and did not reach the expected high values during exercise. In this particular test, it may be possible that the increase in carbohydrate intake associated with a return to normal feeding may have inhibited fat mobilization. Separate studies[25] on biopsy samples have shown that not only is free fatty acid release by adipose tissue enhanced by caloric restriction, but fatty acid synthesis is abolished, so that in the balance, fat tissue would be lost.

On the assumption that rate of fat oxidation is related generally to plasma level of free fatty acid and especially based on Buskirk's[26] findings that obese patients lose more fat when exercise is taken, it can be concluded that obese subjects utilize fats as an energy source during work. Unfortunately, there is a paucity of data defining free fatty acid oxidation rate constants and pool sizes in exercising obese subjects which is necessary in order to arrive at quantitative estimates of fat oxidation during work. Therefore it is not known, with any degree of confidence, whether quantitative extent of fat oxidation is similar in the lean and obese subject for comparable levels of physical work and energy expenditure. Certainly qualitative similarities exist.

Blood glucose metabolism has also been examined in obese subjects under resting conditions. The gross turnover and oxidation rate of glucose in mg/hr is substantially similar in lean and obese subjects despite major body weight differences.[27] In both groups, they decrease during starvation. However, if the extent of glucose metabolism is expressed per kg of body weight, the trend in the obese subject is in the downward direction. Table XI shows the results of tests using labelled glucose. The turnover as shown is a measure of blood glucose replacement (production and release), whereas the oxidation rate is the

TABLE XI

GLUCOSE KINETICS IN NORMAL AND OBESE SUBJECTS
RANGE OF VALUES IS SHOWN

Subjects (No.)	Treatment	Substrate Tested	Turnover Mg/Kg/Hr	Oxidation Mg/Kg/Hr	Ref.
5) Normal	Postabsorptive	Glucose $1C^{14}$	104 - 152.1	--	a
4) Lean	Postabsorptive	Glucose $(UL)C^{14}$	110.3 - 140.6	67.7 - 92.7	b
6) Obese	Postabsorptive	Glucose $1C^{14}$	62.5 - 92.8	--	a
6) Obese	Postabsorptive	Glucose $(UL)C^{14}$	41.1 - 75.7	19.0 - 59.6	b
6) Normal	8 days starvation	Glucose $1C^{14}$	67.1 - 143.0	--	c
2) Lean	7 days starvation	Glucose $1C^{14}$	59.5 - 60.4	40.5 - 40.7	b
4) Obese	7 days starvation	Glucose $1C^{14}$	40 - 93	--	a
2) Obese	5-11 days starvation	Glucose $(UL)C^{14}$	41.3	17.8 - 21.5	b

Kreisberg, R. A. et al. *Diabetes, 19*:53, 1970.
Pavle, P. et al. *Metabolism, 18*:570, 1969.
Cahill, G. F. et al. *J Clin Investigation, 45*:175, 1966.

quantitative estimate of its conversion to CO_2 through oxidative processes. The turnover rate in normal subjects is in the range of 103 to 152 mg/kg/hr and the oxidation rate is 68 to 93 mg/kg/hr. Turnover in the obese subject tends to be lower, 41 to 93 mg/kg/hr, as does the oxidation rate, 19 to 60 mg/kg/hr. During starvation, glucose turnover and oxidation rate is reduced in normal weight subjects; although not entirely clear, the data also suggests a reduction in obese subjects.

Under general resting conditions, a major portion of glucose is oxidized by the central nervous system and to a lesser extent in other body compartments. It is anticipated that those compartments would show similar activities in normal and obese subjects, and that gross oxidation rates without regard to body weight would be similar. Indeed, that was shown to be the case by Paul and Bortz.[27] For this type of evaluation the expression of metabolic data on a fat-free body weight basis may provide a more realistic assessment of glucose metabolism and eliminate some of the apparent ambiguities in the present data base. The present available data suggest that blood glucose turnover and oxidation in obese subjects is close to the normal range.

Although the above data tend to be unclear, other findings suggest a distorted glucose metabolism in overweight subjects. For example, Karam et al.[28] cite evidence that the circulating insulin level rises to a higher level in obese subjects than in normal subjects in response to glucose loading. Despite the high levels of serum insulin in the obese subjects, their blood sugar responses were identical to the normal group. Hence, it was concluded that obese subjects require increased amounts of insulin to maintain normal glucose homeostasis. Jackson and co-workers[29] demonstrated diabetic-like glucose curves in obese subjects with high levels of plasma insulin. Obese patients treated by starvation (seventeen to ninety-nine days) showed improvements in glucose tolerance and a reduction of insulin level; long-term improvements following treatment by food withdrawal showed the therapeutic importance of starvation in the treatment of obesity. Deckert and Hagerup[30] reported serum insulin levels of $28\,\mu$ units/ml in normal weight subjects with no differences in concentration between men and women. Approximately 25 percent of overweight people showed elevated insulin levels. Since none of the subjects with a raised serum insulin level showed a significantly elevated blood sugar, it was concluded on the basis of insulin/glucose ratios that a disturbed blood-sugar regulation existed even though the fasting sugar level was in the normal range. Kreisberg[31] reported that the effect of phenformin HCl, which has an action similar to insulin in increasing peripheral glucose *utilization,* elicits generally similar responses in normal and obese subjects, although the effects on glucose *oxidation* tended to be more variable in the obese. Consequently, responsiveness to insulinlike action was assumed to be similar in the two populations.

With regard to glucose-fat interrelationships, one of the prompt effects of insulin is the enhancement of conversion of glucose to lipid in adipose tissue.[32] The rate of uptake of glucose per gm adipose tissue has been reported to be more or less similar in obese and nonobese subjects.[33] A greater body fat content would thus lead to greater total glucose uptake. The responsiveness of glucose uptake by adipose tissue to exogenous insulin was reduced in obese subjects who were less than 50 percent overweight and absent in subjects more than 50 percent overweight, thus suggesting the development of a resistance in lipogenesis with increasing adiposity. The effect of glucagon which is believed to act directly on the pancreas to give rise to increasing circulating levels of insulin has also been examined.[34] The administration of glucagon in conjunction with glucose resulted in a significantly higher rise in insulin level in obese subjects, although the rate of blood glucose disappearance was not altered significantly. Again, this finding suggests an impaired sensitivity to endogenous insulin in the obese subject.

Compelling evidence for the involvement of insulin in the etiology of obesity and the mechanism of its action is still wanting; the development of a coherent picture of the endocrine mechanisms must await further research. It is worthwhile considering briefly the probable involvement of insulin in exercise and work performance. Searle and Chaikoff[35] made the initial observation that the hyperglycemia induced by glucose infusion induces a transitory cessation of glucose transport from the liver to the blood, an effect mediated possibly by the anticipated rise in serum insulin as a result of the elevated levels of the blood glucose. The administration of insulin alone was later shown[36, 37] to produce a transient inhibition of the release of glucose into the plasma. As discussed in Chapter 2, one characteristic of steady state exercise is a tendency for glucose replacement to rise, and that would be at variance with the effect of insulin. For short periods of exhaustive exercise it has been shown that the insulin level rises as does the blood sugar;[38] but in maximal exercise the contribution of blood glucose oxidation to total caloric expenditure is small. Tests with both normal and diabetic dogs show a lowering of the blood glucose during exercise,[39] presumably through the action of humoral factors *unrelated* to insulin, and the responses could be demonstrated in cross-transfusion experiments. In severe diabetes with a primary insulin insufficiency, the blood glucose replacement rate is apparently substantially higher than normal.[40] In maturity-onset diabetes, exogenous insulin also reduces the blood glucose replacement rate[41] as it does in normal controls.

Insulin depresses the level of plasma free fatty acids under resting conditions[42, 43] and also during exercise.[44] Again, that effect is at variance with the responses observed during work. Thus in the overall balance it would appear that the effect of insulin is antagonistic to some of the key responses to exercise, therefore the participation of or requirement for insulin in exercise is probably negligible or at best debatable.

Returning to the subject of obesity, the studies cited by Albrink[45] suggest that weight gain during adult life rather than obesity per se is associated with hypertriglyceridemia. Men of moderate relative weight, who had then gained additional weight, had higher levels of serum triglycerides than very fat men who had been obese since young manhood. The relationship of triglyceride level to body weight is reasonably well established,[46] and high levels of plasma triglycerides in turn are associated with proneness to coronary atherosclerosis.

The earlier impressive study by Ahrens[47] showed a reduction in serum cholesterol and triglyceride level through the inclusion of unsaturated fats in the diet. Prolonged fasting (17 to 126 days) in uncomplicated obesity produced a significant fall in serum level of triglycerides which was attributed to the exclusion of dietary carbohydrates;[48] conversely, the level of endogenous plasma triglyceride concentration increases with the intake of a high carbohydrate diet.[49] Hyperinsulinemia in the presence of normal to moderately elevated levels of plasma glucose has been suggested as a possible cause of enhanced hepatic triglyceride production by the liver.

In addition to fasting, exercise is also effective in reducing serum triglycerides. Men maintained on an exercise program for several months showed a significant reduction of triglycerides.[50] An analysis of data from the records of 877 flying personnel showed inverse relationships between physical fitness achieved through exercise on the one hand and serum cholesterol and triglyceride level on the other hand.[51] However, the correlations are low and therefore have relatively little predictive value. In healthy subjects participating in competitive skiing events of eight-nine hours duration, the plasma triglycerides are lowered dramatically.[52] Two possible explanations for the acute effects of exercise have been offered: (1) a decreased efflux of triglycerides from the liver to plasma, or (2) an accelerated rate of removal of triglycerides from the plasma.

Dietary studies show that the incorporation of labelled glucose into the serum triglycerides is increased during the intake of a high carbohydrate diet as compared to a high polyunsaturated fat diet,[53] but no consistent differences were noted between hyperglyceridemics and nonhyperglyceridemics. The carbohydrate induced rise in plasma triglyceride concentration has been ascribed to an increased synthesis of triglyceride along with a diminished utilization rate.[54] On the other hand, Ryan and Schwartz[55] proposed that the plasma triglyceride flux rates from the liver are relatively constant and therefore that removal or clearance of the plasma triglycerides is a major determinant of the blood levels. But under general resting conditions[56] as well as during exercise[57] the quantitative removal rate of plasma triglycerides and their oxidation tends to be low, and therefore altered plasma clearance rate would not seem to be a likely factor contributing to rapid changes in blood levels.

In order to clarify the acute effects of exercise, healthy postabsorptive subjects were studied during a thirteen and one half hour period of either rest or treadmill walking. During the latter four and one half hour period of testing, uniformly labelled substrates were administered intravenously and their incorporation into plasma triglycerides was determined. During several hours of rest, the average level of serum triglyceride was 64 mg/100 ml; during exercise, the level was 40 mg/100 ml. The time history of incorporation is shown in Figure 7. In general, the curves for resting and exercising subjects tend to overlay each other in terms of the time history of the response, and therefore the dynamics which regulate the rise and fall of the labelled triglycerides are similar in both groups. On the other hand, the activity incorporated is less during exercise and this argues strongly for a reduced hepatic triglyceride synthesis and secretion rate or a reduced uptake of substrates by the liver during exercise. Whether those same mechanisms are operant

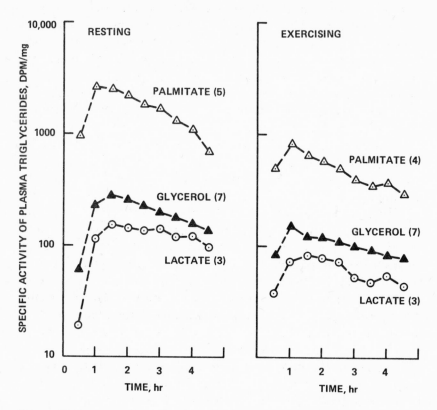

Figure 7. Incorporation of ¹⁴C uniformly labelled substrates (palmitate, glycerol, lactate) into circulating plasma triglycerides after nine hours of rest or exercise. Specific activity of plasma triglycerides in DPM/mg is shown on the vertical scale; time following IV administration of substrates is shown on the horizontal scale. Number of subjects is shown in parentheses.

to reduce plasma triglyceride level as a result of reducing carbohydrate, or during food deprivation in the obese, or are an exclusive result of physical fitness programs is not known. Nevertheless, a reduction in synthesis rate seems a reasonable explanation.

In general, the overweight subject shows a number of similarities to the normal population with regard to the responses to diet and exercise. If large quantitative differences exist, they are difficult to demonstrate because of the problem of evaluating, equivalently, the obese and lean. Clearly, energy expenditure and the physiologic cost of work is mass related and related to state of physical fitness. Type and quantity of body tissue lost during food restriction are similar in both groups.

REFERENCES

1. Bloom, W. L. and Eidex, M. F.: The comparison of energy expenditure in the obese and lean. *Metabolism, 16*:685-692, 1967.
2. Åstrand, I., Åstrand, P., and Stunkard, A.: Oxygen intake of obese individuals during work on a bicycle ergometer. *Acta Physiol Scand, 50*:294-299, 1960.
3. Buskirk, E. and Taylor, H. L.: Maximal oxygen intake and its relation to body composition. With special reference to chronic physical activity and obesity. *J Appl Physiol, 11*:72-78, 1957.
4. Young, D. R.: Effect of body composition and weight gain on performance in the adult dog. *J Appl Physiol, 15*:493-495, 1960.
5. Young, D. R., Mosher, R., Erve, P., and Spector, H.: Energy metabolism and gas exchange during treadmill running in dogs. *J Appl Physiol, 14*:834-838, 1959.
6. Carlson, L. A. and Fröberg, S. O.: Blood lipid and glucose levels during a ten-day period of low-calorie intake and exercise in man. *Metabolism, 16*:624-634, 1967.
7. Young, D. R.: Effect of food deprivation on treadmill running in dogs. *J Appl Physiol, 14*:1018-1022, 1959.
8. Buskirk, E. R., Thompson, R. H., Lutwak, L., and Whedon, G. D.: Energy balance of obese patients during weight reduction: Influence of diet restriction and exercise. *Ann N Y Acad Sci, 110*:918-940, 1963.
9. Issekutz, B., Bortz, W. M., Miller, H. I., and Wroldsen, A.: Plasma free fatty acid response to exercise in obese humans. *Metabolism, 16*:492-502, 1967.
10. Consolazio, C. F., Matoush, O., Johnson, H. L., Nelson, R. A., and Krzywick, H. J.: Metabolic aspects of acute starvation in normal humans (10 days). *Am J Clin Nutr, 20*:672-683, 1967.
11. Benoit, F. L., Martin, R. L., and Watten, R. H.: Changes in body composition during weight reduction in obesity. Balance studies comparing effects of fasting and a ketogenic diet. *Ann Intern Med, 63*:604-612, 1965.
12. Berlin, N. I., Watkins, D. M., and Gervitz, N. R.: Measurement of changes in gross body composition during controlled weight reduction in obesity by metabolic balance and body density. Body water technics. *Metabolism, 11*:302-314, 1962.
13. Birkenhager, J. C., Haak, A., and Ackers, J. G.: Changes in body composition during treatment of obesity by intermittent starvation. *Metabolism, 17*:391-399, 1968.
14. Ball, M. F., Canary, J. J., and Kyle, L. H.: Comparative effects of caloric

restriction and total starvation on body composition in obesity. *Ann Intern Med, 67*:60-67, 1967.
15. Benoit, Martin, and Watten: Changes in body composition.
16. Grande, F.: Energy balance and body composition changes. A critical study of three recent publications. *Ann Intern Med, 68*:467-480, 1968.
17. Buskirk et al.: Energy balance.
18. Buskirk et al.: Energy balance.
19. Gordon, E. S.: Non-esterified fatty acids in the blood of obese and lean subjects. *Am J Clin Nutr, 8*:740-747, 1960.
20. Goldberg, M. and Gordon, E. S.: Energy metabolism in human obesity. *JAMA, 189*:104-123, 1964.
21. Gordon, E. S. and Goldberg, M.: Studies of energy metabolism in human subjects using carbon 14-labeled compounds. I. Effect of sex, state of nutrition and body weight. *Metabolism, 13*:775-790, 1964.
22. Brown, J.: Metabolism of free fatty acids in obese humans. *Proc Soc Exp Biol Med, 110*:901-904, 1962.
23. Issekutz, B., Pavle, P., Miller, H. I., and Bortz, W. M.: Oxidation of plasma FFA in lean and obese humans. *Metabolism, 17*:62-73, 1968.
24. Issekutz, B., Bortz, W. M., Miller, H. I., and Wroldsen, A.: Plasma free fatty acid response to exercise in obese humans. *Metabolism, 16*:492-502, 1967.
25. Goldrick, R. B. and Hirsch, J.: Serial studies on the metabolism of human adipose tissue. II. Effects of caloric restriction and refeeding on lipogenesis, and the uptake and release of free fatty acids in obese and nonobese individuals. *J Clin Invest, 43*:1793-1804, 1964.
26. Buskirk et al.: Energy balance.
27. Paul, P. and Bortz, W. M.: Turnover and oxidation of plasma glucose in lean and obese subjects. *Metabolism, 18*:570-584, 1969.
28. Karam, J. H., Grodsky, G. M., and Forsham, P. H.: Excessive insulin response to glucose in obese subjects as measured by immunochemical assay. *Diabetes, 12*:197-204, 1963.
29. Jackson, I. M. D., McKiddie, M. T., and Buchanan, K. D.: The effect of fasting on glucose and insulin metabolism of obese patients. *Lancet, 7509*:285-287, Jan. 1969.
30. Deckert, T. and Hagerup, L.: Serum insulin in normal and obese persons. *Acta Med Scand, 182*:225-232, 1967.
31. Kreisberg, R. A.: Glucose metabolism in normal and obese subjects. *Diabetes, 17*:481-488, 1968.
32. Mellati, A. M., Beck, J. C., Dupre, J., and Rubinstein, D.: Conversion of glucose to lipid by human adipose tissue *in vitro*. *Metabolism, 19*:988-994, 1970.
33. Englhardt, A., Kasperek, R., Liebermeister, H., and Jahnke, K.: Studies glucose utilization and insulin responsiveness of human subcutaneous adipose tissue in obese and nonobese subjects. *Horm Metab Res, 3*:266-272, 1971.

34. Benedetti, A., Simpson, R. G., Grodsky, G. M., and Forsham, P. H.: Exaggerated insulin response to glucagon in simple obesity. *Diabetes, 16:*666-669, 1967.

35. Searle, G. L. and Chaikoff, I. L.: Inhibitory action of hyperglycemia on delivery of glucose to the blood stream by the liver of the normal dog. *Am J Physiol, 170:*456-460, 1952.

36. Searle, G. L., Mortimore, G. E., Buckley, R. E., and Reilly, W. A.: Plasma glucose turnover in humans as studied with C¹⁴ glucose. Influence of insulin and tolbutamide. *Diabetes, 8:*167-173, 1959.

37. Craig, J. W., Drucker, W. R., Miller, M., and Woodward, H.: A prompt effect of exogenous insulin on net hepatic glucose output in man. *Metabolism, 10:*212-220, 1961.

38. Hermansen, L., Pruett, E. D. R., Osnes, J. B., and Giere, F. A.: Blood glucose and plasma insulin in response to maximal exercise and glucose infusion. *J Appl Physiol, 29:*13-16, 1970.

39. Goldstein, M. S.: Humoral nature of hypoglycemia in muscular exercise. *Am J Physiol, 200:*67-70, 1961.

40. Reichard, G. A., Jr., Jacobs, A. G., Kimbel, P., Hochella, N. J., and Weinhouse, S.: Blood glucose replacement rates in normal and diabetic humans. *J Appl Physiol, 16:*789-795, 1961.

41. Kalant, N., Csorba, T. R., and Heller, N.: Effect of insulin on glucose production and utilization in diabetes. *Metabolism, 12:*1100-1111, 1963.

42. Burns, T. W., Gehrke, C. W., and Anigian, M. J.: Effect of insulin on plasma free fatty acids of normal subjects. *J Lab Clin Med, 62:*646-656, 1963.

43. Shreeve, W. W.: Effects of insulin on the turnover of plasma carbohydrates and lipids. *Am J Med, 40:*724-734, 1966.

44. Shapiro, J., Young, D. R., Datnow, B., and Pelligra, R.: Development of a standard prolonged work test for the evaluation of fatigue and stress in man. *Aerospace Med, 38:*268-272, 1967.

45. Albrink, M. J.: Triglycerides, lipoproteins, and coronary artery disease. *Arch Intern Med, 109:*345-359, 1962.

46. Hollister, L. E., Overall, J. E., and Snow, H. L.: Relationship of obesity to serum triglyceride, cholesterol, and uric acid, and to plasma-glucose levels. *Am J Clin Nutr, 20:*777-782, 1967.

47. Ahrens, E. H., Hirsch, J., Insull, W., Tsaltas, T. T., Blomstrand, R., and Peterson, M. L.: The influence of dietary fats on serum-lipid levels in man. *Lancet, 1,* Issue No. *6976:*943-953, 1957.

48. Jackson, I. M. D.: Effect of prolonged starvation on blood lipid levels of obese subjects. *Metabolism, 18:*13-17, 1969.

49. Farquhar, J. W., Frank, A., Gross, R. C., and Reaven, G. M.: Glucose, insulin, and triglyceride responses to high and low carbohydrate diets in man. *J Clin Invest, 45:*1648-1656, 1966.

50. Holloszy, J. O., Skinner, J. S., Toro, G., and Cureton, T. K.: Effects of a six-month program of endurance exercise on the serum lipids of

middle-aged men. *Am J Cardiol, 14:*753-757, 1964.
51. Shane, S. R.: Relation between serum lipids and physical conditioning. *Am J Cardiol, 18:*540-543, 1966.
52. Carlson, L. A. and Mossfeldt, F.: Acute effects of prolonged, heavy exercise on the concentration of plasma lipids and lipoproteins in man. *Acta Physiol Scand, 62:*51-59, 1964.
53. Fine, M., Michaels, G., Shah, S., Chai, B., Fukayama, G., and Kinsell, L.: The incorporation of C^{14} from uniformly labeled glucose into plasma triglycerides in normals and hyperglyceridemics. *Metabolism, 11:*893-910, 1962.
54. Nestel, P. J. and Hirsch, E. Z.: Triglyceride turnover after diets rich in carbohydrate or animal fat. *Aust Ann Med, 14:*265-269, 1965.
55. Ryan, W. G. and Schwartz, T. B.: Dynamics of plasma triglyceride turnover in man. *Metabolism, 14:*1243-1254, 1965.
56. Farquhar, J. W., Gross, R. C., Wagner, R. M., and Reaven, G. M.: Validation of an incompletely coupled two-compartment nonrecycling catenary model for turnover of liver and plasma triglyceride in man. *J Lipid Res, 6:*119-134, 1965.
57. Young, D. R., Shapira, J., Forrest, R., Adachi, R. R., Lim, R., and Pelligra, R.: Model for evaluation of fatty acid metabolism for man during prolonged exercise. *J Appl Physiol, 23:*716-725, 1967.

Chapter 4

GROWTH HORMONE AND
INSULIN MECHANISMS

So far, emphasis has been placed upon carbohydrate and fat metabolism with respect to exercise and different nutritional and health states. Growth hormone has been implicated as one of the factors associated with glucose output by the liver as well as lipolysis. The biochemical details of fatty acid metabolism as well as the dynamic balance in blood sugar regulation have been reviewed in considerable detail[1, 2] and will not be covered here.

Given that growth hormone is one factor in a multiplicity and hierarchy of controlling phenomena in liver glucose production, it is pertinent to inquire into some of the operating and performance features of the system, and in particular the mechanisms which regulate the release of growth hormone from the pituitary. In the absence of complete data, adequate sampling techniques, etc., biological modelling is a useful procedure not only as an analysis technique to attempt to predict observed responses, but also to elucidate delicate and difficult points of theory. *Ad hoc* models of biological systems are not simply a tour de force in the solution of differential equations; rather, they attempt to describe and evaluate a process symbolically and deductively. Importantly, they also attempt to seek generalizations which may point to promising new leads in research. Thus, even though models may be only caricatures of reality, if they are minimally adequate they will also portray some of the features of the real biological system. Recent pioneers in the development of models of glucose homeostasis are Bolie,[3] Ceresa et al.,[4] and Janes and Osburn[5] who evaluated insulin-glucose interactions and Ackerman et al.[6] who extended the evaluations to include growth hormone effects.

The early literature citing the effects of growth hormone on carbohydrate metabolism has been reviewed by DeBodo and Altszuler.[7] Selected references from that review demonstrate (1) a depressed hepatic glucose output in hypophysectomized animals, (2) that in hypophysectomized animals maintained on a daily growth hormone regimen, the rate of flow of glucose from the liver into the plasma increases, (3) that large doses of growth hormone can produce glycosuria and diabetes in experimental animals, and (4) that replacement therapy of growth hormone in hypophysectomized animals ameliorates or abolishes insulin hypersensitivity. Luft and Cerasi[8] reviewed several of the studies following the availability in 1956 of human growth hormone for tests in man. The demonstration in 1960 that human growth hormone could induce a transient diabetic state in human subjects provided the evidence for ascribing to growth hormone the role of a significant diabetogenic factor in man. The authors cite evidence that a decrease in blood glucose of at least 10 mg percent is accompanied by a rise in plasma growth hormone generally in proportion to the degree of hypoglycemia.

The data form the basis for postulating a preliminary regulatory system involving level of blood glucose, pituitary growth hormone production, and hepatic glucose production. Further evidence in support of the concept of a closed loop regulatory system is provided by the following observations: (1) a decrease in blood glucose is a stimulus for additional growth hormone secretion;[9, 10] (2) the level of serum growth hormone is elevated during physical exercise;[11, 12, 13, 14] (3) growth hormone releasing factor is secreted apparently by the hypothalamus and transported to the anterior pituitary by means of the microcirculation of the brain;[15] (4) growth hormone released by the pituitary is transported in the circulation to tissues such as the liver which are known to have a high rate of glucose production; (5) the level of blood growth hormone tends to regulate the secretion rate from the pituitary;[16] (6) the level of blood glucose regulates the secretion of glucose by the liver.[17] Based upon the available data, a conceptual model of blood glucose regulation involving only growth hormone can be formulated as shown in Figure 8.

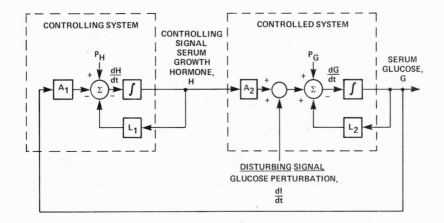

Figure 8. Model for the evaluation of glucose regulation in postabsorptive subjects. (Young, D. R., et al. *Comp Biomed Res, 3*:74, 1970.)

Insofar as growth hormone may be a regulator of carbohydrate metabolism during exercise when glucose production and oxidation increase, attempts have been made to uncover some of the possible mechanisms modifying its secretion rate from the pituitary in relationship to level of physical activity. In order to determine the limits of validity of the proposed model, the evaluation has been extended to include the condition of sleep, which from an energy expenditure point of view is at the lower end of the energy cost continuum. The major assumptions in modelling are as follows: (1) each regulatory organ system functions as a reservoir for growth hormone or glucose and as a detector for the respective compounds; (2) growth hormone and glucose are lost from the plasma at various rates, depending upon the physiologic state of other tissues, and the losses are interpreted as loads upon the controller and controlled system; (3) irregularities in plasma mixing dynamics are ignored; and (4) reserves and precursor materials for growth hormone or glucose biosynthesis are not rate limiting factors in normal regulation.

In order to evaluate the kinetic response of the serum growth hormone level, experiments were conducted with seven postabsorptive subjects studied during a twelve-hour period of exercise or rest. Insulin was administered intravenously to depress

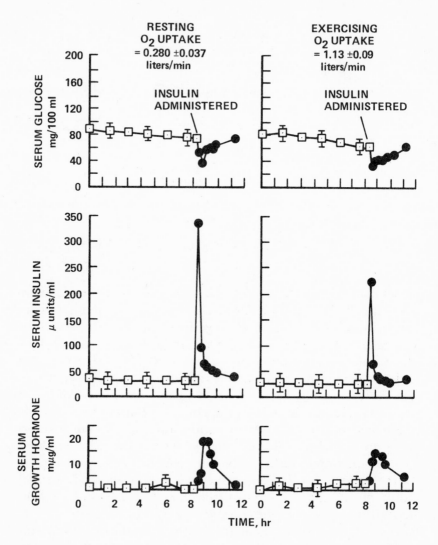

Figure 9. Serum growth hormone response following the administration of IV insulin to resting or exercising subjects. Serum concentration of glucose, insulin, and growth hormone is shown on the vertical axis; test duration in hr is shown on the horizontal axis. (Young, D. R., et al. *Comp Biomed Res,* 3:74, 1970.)

the level of blood glucose and the time history of the serum growth hormone response was determined. The data upon which the model was tested are shown in Figure 9. Symbols and definitions developed in the study are shown in Table XII.

TABLE XII

NOTATIONS FOR SERUM GROWTH HORMONE MODEL

Symbol	Definition	Dimensions
a	Parameter which determines the rate of growth	$1/\text{min}$
a_1	Sensitivity of serum growth hormone production to serum glucose concentration	$\dfrac{m\mu g H/ml/min}{mg\ G/ml}$
a_2	Sensitivity of serum glucose production to serum growth hormone concentration	$\dfrac{mg\ G/ml/min}{m\mu g\ H/ml}$
G	Serum glucose concentration	mg/ml
H	Serum growth hormone concentration	$m\mu g/ml$
H_C	Command signal for growth hormone production	
H_F	Final steady-state value of serum growth hormone	$m\mu g/ml$
H_f	Feedback level of growth hormone	$m\mu g/ml$
H_p	Peak value of serum growth hormone	$m\mu g/ml$
H_{ss}	Steady-state value of serum growth hormone	$m\mu g/ml$
I	Time history of glucose perturbation	mg/ml
l_1	Sensitivity of growth hormone production to growth hormone concentration	$1/\text{min}$
l_2	Sensitivity of glucose production to glucose concentration	$1/\text{min}$
$l_2 p_H - a_1 p_G$	Parameter which determines final steady-state values of serum growth hormone concentration	$m\mu g/ml$
P_G	Production rate of glucose per unit volume of serum	$mg/ml/min$
P_H	Production rate of growth hormone per unit volume of serum	$m\mu g/ml/min$
s	Laplace transform exponent	
T	Period of oscillation	min
k	Integer	

Briefly, during eight and one fourth hours of exercise, the level of serum glucose declined from 84 to 68 mg percent and the level of growth hormone increased from 0.70 to 2.9 $m\mu g/ml$. Following the administration of insulin, the serum glucose declined to 38 mg percent and then returned slowly to preinjection levels; after a slight delay the level of serum growth hormone rose to 14.4 $m\mu g/ml$ and then returned toward preinjection levels.

During resting conditions, the level of serum glucose declined from 89 to 76 mg percent. The level of serum growth hormone was relatively constant, 0.60 mμg/ml. Subsequent to the administration of insulin, the level of serum glucose declined to 39 mg percent and then returned to preinjection levels; the level of serum growth hormone rose to 18.3 mμg/ml and then declined.

When the relationships shown in Figure 8 are expressed in mathematical form, the following first order differential equations are obtained:

$$dG/dt = pG - l_2G + a_2H + dI/dt \qquad [1]$$
$$dH/dt = pH - l_1H - a_1G \qquad [2]$$

The inclusion of p_G and p_H is based upon the reported endogenous production of glucose by the liver[18] and growth hormone production by pituitary explants.[19] Solving the equations for serum growth hormone concentration, H, and assuming the growth hormone response to be critically damped provides the following relationship:

$$\frac{d^2H}{dt^2} + \frac{2adH}{dt} + a^2(H) = (l_2p_H - a_1\, p_G) - a_1\frac{(dI)}{(dt)} \qquad [3]$$

Where $(l_1 + l_2) = 2a$ [4]
and $(l_1l_2 + a_1a_2) = a^2$ [5]

where "a" determines the rate of rise and fall of serum growth hormone, "a_1" represents the sensitivity of growth hormone production rate to glucose concentration and is considered to be an amplification factor. The term dI/dt is the rate of change of glucose and is the forcing function giving rise to the growth hormone response. The parameter $(l_2\, p_H - a_1\, p_G)$ is related to the final values of H following the perturbation.

The serum growth hormone responses of resting and working subjects are shown in Figures 10 and 11. Good agreements are found between observed and computed values. Computed values for the parameter "a" are 0.0045 and 0.0078 for exercising and resting conditions, respectively. The computed value for "a_1" is 2.3 for both conditions of exercise and rest.

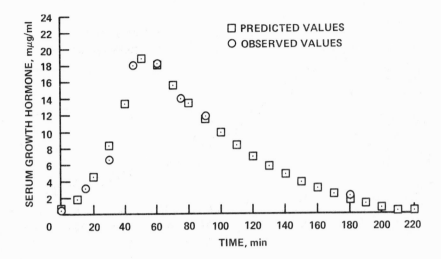

Figure 10. Serum growth hormone response to IV insulin in *resting* subjects. Growth hormone level in mg/ml is shown on the vertical axis; test duration in min is shown on the horizontal scale. Observed values are shown with the open circles; predicted values with the parameter 0.0078 are shown with the open squares. (Young, D. R., et al. *Comp Biomed Res*, *3*:74, 1970.)

When the parameter "a" is greater than its nominal value, the response is reduced.

If an open-loop condition were produced, that is, a relative dissociation or uncoupling of the pituitary from the level of blood glucose, the response of the pituitary would depend on the relative magnitude of the two system parameters. For example, the model predicts that if $a_1 = 2a$ the secretory response of the pituitary would be oscillatory and would be very lightly damped. Furthermore, values of a_1 small enough to satisfy the equality would virtually isolate the pituitary gland from the glucose environment and therefore the amplitude of the oscillation would be very small unless a new and higher steady-state or reference growth hormone level were established.

Sleep is an interesting physiologic phenomenon which apparently decouples the pituitary from the glucose environment. The serum growth hormone level during sleep was measured experimentally by Takahashi et al.[20] Their results show that during the initial stages of deep sleep the pituitary secretion of growth hormone shows an undamped oscillation with a period

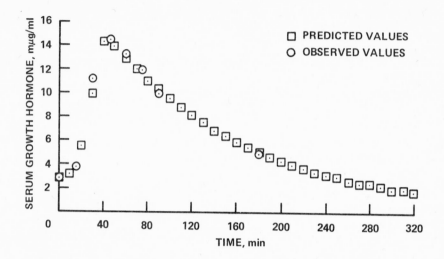

Figure 11. Serum growth hormone response to IV insulin in *exercising* subjects. Observed values are shown with the open circles. Predicted values with the parameter 0.0045 are shown with the open squares. (Young, D. R., et al. *Comp Biomed Res, 3*:74, 1970.)

of approximately three and one half hours. Accordingly, the model parameters are,

$$a = 2\pi/T = 0.03$$
$$\text{and, } a_1 = 2a = 0.06$$

This supports the concept that the glandular mechanism is operating as an open-loop system during the initial phase of sleep. Furthermore, the level of blood hormone is increased to a value equal to the amplitude of the hormonal response plus the new steady state value. At the termination of one oscillation (one cycle), normal operation is restored. The mathematical details of the development and formulation of the time history response of the pituitary, operating in the open-loop mode, have been presented elsewhere[21] and will not be covered here. However, the results are shown in Table XIII and Figures 12, 13, and 14, where it can be seen that there is good agreement between experimental and theoretical results. It is important to note that this analysis is predicated on the relative loss of control and regulation of pituitary secretions. The good conformation between experimental data and predicted responses indicates that it is a good first order approximation of the regulatory system.

TABLE XIII

	Time		Growth Hormone Concentration, (Ht) mμg/ml						
k	*kT/8*	*Minutes*	H_p 18.0	H_{ss} 1.0	H_p 24.0	H_{ss} 2.0	H_p 40.0	H_{ss} 4.0	H_p 48.0 H_{ss} 2.0
0	0	0	1.00		2.00		4.00		2.00
1	T/8	26.25	3.49		5.23		9.27		8.74
2	T/4	52.50	9.50		13.00		22.00		25.00
3	3T/8	78.75	15.51		20.80		34.74		41.27
4	T/2	105.00	18.00		24.00		40.00		48.00
5	5T/8	131.25	15.51		20.80		34.74		41.27
6	3T/4	157.50	9.50		13.00		22.00		25.00
7	7T/8	183.75	3.49		5.23		9.27		8.74
8	T	210.00	1.00		2.00		4.00		2.00

The results of Takahashi show that the amplitudes of the oscillations induced during the initial phase of sleep varies from 8.5 to 23 mμg/ml. The time history of the response, H(t), shown here was evaluated at intervals of T/8.

From: Howard, J. C. and Young, D. R. *Indian J Nutr Diet, 11*:144-168, 1974.

With respect to the body's ability to maintain the blood glucose within limits as a result of complex interactions between carbohydrate, precursors of carbohydrate, and various hormones, the above analysis and evaluation suggests that: (1) Somewhere in the body there exists a functional glucose sensor; (2) This sensor is sensitive and reactive to rates of change in the blood glucose level; (3) Information regarding the glucose environment is transmitted to the pituitary, undergoes gain or amplification, and is a determinant in the quantity of growth hormone secreted; (4) Both the sensitivity of the pituitary gland's growth hormone production rate to serum growth hormone concentration, and the sensitivity of the body's glucose production rate to serum glucose concentration determine the rise and fall in the blood level of growth hormone; when these

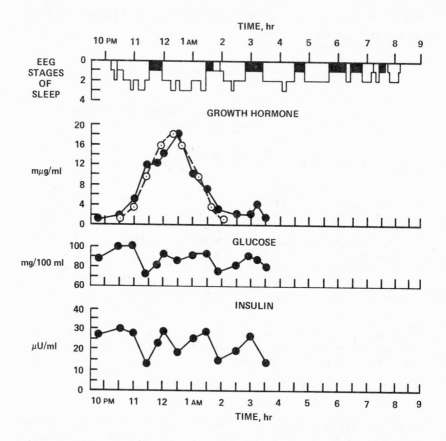

Figure 12. Serum growth hormone, glucose, and insulin during a normal night's sleep in a twenty-seven-year-old man. The level of sleep is indicated at the top; the cross-hatched areas are periods of rapid eye movement. Time of day is shown on the horizontal scale. Predicted values of growth hormone are shown by the open circles. (Howard, J. C. and Young, D. R. *Indian J Nutr Diet, 11*:144, 1974.)

sensitivities are greater than nominal values, not only is the peak amplitude of the hormonal response diminished but the blood levels are attenuated sooner; and (5) Deep sleep apparently decouples the pituitary gland from the blood level of glucose and the sensitivity of growth hormone production to glucose concentration, reflected in the numerical value of "a_1" is reduced to such an extent that the pituitary feedback loop is deactivated and open-loop operation prevails for several hours.

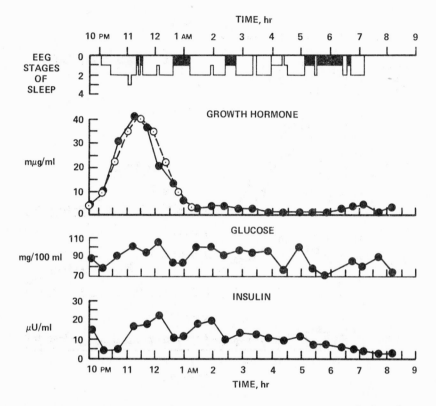

Figure 13. Reproducibility of serum growth hormone response during sleep. This control study was carried out on the same individual as shown in Figure 12. Predicted values for growth hormone are shown by the open circles. (Howard, J. C. and Young, D. R. *Indian J Nutr Diet, 11*:144, 1974.)

One possible model of the control system is shown in Figure 15.

Implications from the model follow. (1) During physical activity, the release of growth hormone from the pituitary is proportional to rate of change and magnitude of depression of the blood glucose. (2) The flow of hepatic glucose into the blood is in part regulated by the serum level of growth hormone in order to assure a production and release rate of glucose consistent with the metabolic demand and requirements. (3) With decreasing levels of physical activity, growth hormone secretion is controlled and regulated to a lesser extent by the

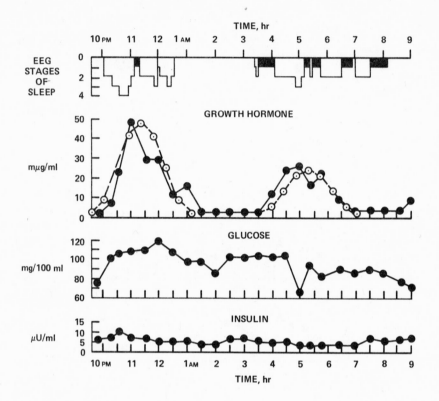

Figure 14. Effect of interruption of sleep (3 hr) on the serum growth hormone response. Predicted values of growth hormone are shown by the open circles. (Howard, J. C. and Young, D. R. *Indian J Nutr Diet, 11*:144, 1974.)

serum glucose, until finally in deep sleep the sensitivities for crosscoupling are so reduced that the pituitary secretions are relatively independent of blood glucose levels. (4) One of the sensitivity coefficients that determines the rate of increased secretions of growth hormone is closely related to activity level in that it is larger in resting subjects than in exercising subjects and is still larger in subjects who are in a state of deep sleep. Thus, the latter parameter is specific for physical exercise and trends of caloric expenditure.

The foregoing analysis serves a heuristic function in identifying future experiment requirements. For example, promising areas of research would include investigations into the mechan-

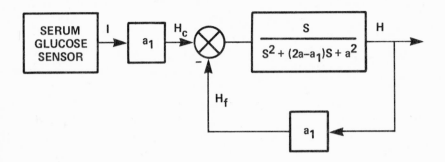

Figure 15. Model of a growth hormone control system with feedback gain.

isms of information transfer and flow between the pituitary and serum glucose and the effects of wakefulness, activity level, and psychomotor stimulants such as imipramine[22] which tend to abolish the serum oscillations of growth hormone level.

Although growth hormone appears to be an important regulatory factor in carbohydrate metabolism during exercise, its relatedness to altered nutritional states is much less documented. During short periods of food deprivation (one to three days), the blood level of growth hormone increases and the blood glucose level declines.[23] Prolonged food deprivation which may produce a panhypopituitarism could alter the regulatory function of the pituitary. The evidence cited in Chapter 3 showing reductions in blood glucose replacement rate during fasting may have, as an underlying basis, disruptions in the homeostatic feedback system.

Insulin has been viewed as another controller of the flow of stored body fuels. That is, high levels of insulin are associated with the *fed* state, low levels are associated with *fasting*, and the flow of substrates between tissue storage and mobilization is determined by the controller. For example, the maintenance of the blood glucose between meals is probably supported for the most part by glycogenolysis and the release of glucose from the liver. In one particular series of tests, Long and coworkers[24] estimated liver glucose production to be approximately 125 mg/min; infusion of exogenous glucose at that rate brought about a prompt cessation of liver glucose production. An explanation for that response proposed by Cahill[25] is that the pancreatic *receptors* are extremely sensitive to inputs of glucose, perceiving small differences in glucose levels, and releasing insulin which in turn suppresses liver glucose output. In any event, it demonstrates the autoregulation between blood levels of glucose and liver carbohydrate production. In the event that large excursions of the blood glucose occur such as following carbohydrate meals, released insulin increases the rate of disposal of the blood glucose; approximately 40 percent flows to muscle glycogen, 25 percent is converted into fat, 10 percent is transformed into liver glycogen, and the remainder is oxidized.

The evidence presented in Chapter 3 suggests a possible relationship between insulin and glucose in obesity. The disposition of glucose in peripheral tissue and in particular its conversion to lipids was thought originally to serve as a focus for a unifying theory in fat synthesis and storage. Not only does elevated level of blood insulin increase the conversion of glucose to lipid, it also promotes the uptake of chilomicrons and neutral fats through the activation of lipoprotein lipase. Therefore, additional observations relevant to insulin responses in obesity are worth noting. Unfortunately, the data tend to be largely descriptive and insufficient for the formulation of a preliminary control system model. Karam and co-workers[26, 27] demonstrated that obese subjects as a group responded to glucose loading with excessive blood insulin levels and therefore raised the possibility that adiposity per se influences the plasma insulin response. Critical tests of that hypothesis were undertaken by Perley and Kipnis.[28, 29] The plasma insulin response to oral glucose was threefold greater in obese subjects; insulin secretion following intravenous tolbutamide was fourfold greater in obese subjects. The authors concluded that obesity was associated with a hypersecretory insulin response. Obese subjects show high levels of endogenous plasma insulin[30] under fasting conditions, and high levels during the glucose tolerance test.[31] Additional factors may be associated with insulin secretion; factors such as epinephrine have been shown to inhibit pancreatic insulin release,[32] and growth hormone apparently increases the synthesis and secretion of insulin.[33, 34]

In untreated acromegalics and also in obese subjects tested during IV insulin administration, the blood glucose at first declines, then returns towards preinjection levels more rapidly than in normal subjects.[35] This has been interpreted as demonstrating a resistance to insulin due to elevated blood growth hormone levels. However, under general resting conditions, the acromegalic shows a normal rate of glucose oxidation which accounts for approximately 50 percent of the glucose turnover per unit time;[36] perhaps the disposition of the remainder, whether flow to glycogen or fat, could differ from normals.

What appears to emerge from the data is that the obese subject shows a hypersecretion of insulin particularly in the presence of a glucose disturbance. Although the amplitude of the serum insulin response is greater than normal, the time history in terms of the rise and decline of insulin does not appear to be importantly different. Slightly greater glucose loads are required in the obese subject in order to reproduce the normal blood glucose curve and profile[37] and that indicates in addition a different rate of disposal of glucose. One controlling factor is blood level of insulin which stimulates lipogenesis from glucose. Whether growth hormone in those subjects makes available additional quantities of glucose is uncertain. Adipose tissue itself shows a degree of autoregulation in that lipogenesis per unit mass of tissue is reduced in the grossly obese subject. Whether or not this is due to intrinsic factors within the cell, extrinsic factors, or ratios of cell surfaces to volume, i.e. number of cells, is unknown.

REFERENCES

1. Fritz, I. B.: Factors influencing the rates of long-chain fatty acid oxidation and synthesis in mammalian systems. *Physiol Rev, 41*:52-129, 1961.
2. Soskin, S.: The blood sugar: Its origin, regulation and utilization. *Physiol Rev, 21*:140-193, 1941.
3. Bolie, V. W.: Coefficients of normal blood glucose regulation. *J Appl Physiol, 16*:783-788, 1961.
4. Ceresa, F., Ghemi, F., Martini, P. F., Martino, P., Segre, G., and Vitelli, A.: Control of blood glucose in normal and in diabetic subjects. Studies by compartmental analysis and digital computer technics.

84   *Physical Performance, Fitness, and Diet*

Diabetes, 17:570-578, 1968.
5. Janes, R. G. and Osburn, J. O.: The analysis of glucose measurements by computer simulation. *J Physiol, 181*:59-67, 1965.
6. Ackerman, E., Gatewood, L. C., Rosevear, J. W., and Molnar, G. D.: Model studies of blood glucose regulation. *Bull Math Biophys, 27*:21-37, 1965.
7. DeBodo, R. C. and Altszuler, N.: Insulin hypersensitivity and physiological insulin antagonists. *Physiol Rev, 38*:389-445, 1958.
8. Luft, R. and Cerasi, E.: Human growth hormone as a regulator of blood glucose concentration and as a diabetogenic substance. *Acta Endocrinol, (Suppl), 124*:9-16, 1967.
9. Roth, J., Glick, S. M., Yalow, R. S., and Berson, S. A.: The influence of blood glucose on the plasma concentration of growth hormone. *Diabetes, 13*:355-361, 1964.
10. Roth, J., Glick, S. M., Yalow, R. S., and Berson, S. A.: Hypoglycemia: a potent stimulus to secretion of growth hormone. *Science, 140*:987-988, 1963.
11. Roth et al.: Influence of blood glucose.
12. Hunter, W. M., Fonsenka, C. C., and Passmore, R.: Growth hormone: Important role in muscular exercise in adults. *Science, 150*:1051-1053, 1965.
13. Roth, J., Glick, S. M., Yalow, R. S., and Berson, S. A.: Secretion of human growth hormone: Physiologic and experimental modification. *Metabolism, 12*:577-579, 1963.
14. Schalch, D. S.: The influence of physical stress and exercise on growth hormone and insulin secretion in man. *J Lab Clin Med, 69*:256-269, 1967.
15. Müller, E. E., Arimura, A., Sawano, S., Saito, T., and Schally, A. V.: Growth hormone-releasing activity in the hypothalamus and plasma of rats subjected to stress. *Proc Soc Exp Biol Med, 125*:874-878, 1967.
16. Müller, E. E., Sawano, S., Arimura, A., and Schally, A. V.: Mechanism of action of growth hormone in altering its own secretion rate: Comparison with the action of dexamethasone. *Acta Endocrinol, 56*:499-509, 1967.
17. Glinsmann, W. H., Hern, E. P., and Lynch, A.: Intrinsic regulation of glucose output by rat liver. *Am J Physiol, 216*:698-703, 1969.
18. Wagle, S. R., Gaskins, P. K., Jacoby, A., and Ashmore, J.: Studies on glucose synthesis by rat liver and kidney cortex slices. *Life Sci, 6*:655-663, 1966.
19. Birge, C. A., Peake, G. T., Mariz, I. K., and Daughaday, W. H.: Effects of cortisol and diethylstilbesterol on growth hormone release by rat pituitary *in vitro*. *Proc Soc Exp Biol Med, 126*:342-345, 1967.
20. Takahashi, Y., Kipnis, D. M., and Daughaday, W. H.: Growth hormone secretion during sleep. *J Clin Invest, 47*:2079-2090, 1968.
21. Howard, J. C. and Young, D. R.: A simplified control system for

predicting the hypophyseal, growth hormone response of human subjects to various physical activities. *Indian J Nutr Diet, 11*:144-168, 1974.

22. Takahashi et al.: Growth hormone secretion during sleep.
23. Misbin, R. I., Edgar, P. J., and Lockwood, D. H.: Influence of adrenergic receptor stimulation on glucose metabolism during starvation in man: effects on circulating levels of insulin growth hormone and free fatty acid. *Metabolism, 20*:544-554, 1971.
24. Long, C. L., Spencer, J. L., Kinney, J. N., and Geiger, J. W.: Carbohydrate metabolism in normal man and effect of glucose infusion. *J Appl Physiol, 31*:102-109, 1971.
25. Cahill, G. F.: Physiology of insulin in man. *Diabetes, 20*:785-799, 1971.
26. Karam, J. H., Pavlatos, F. C., Grodsky, G. M., and Fordsham, P. H.: Critical factors in excessive serum-insulin response to glucose. *Lancet, 1*:286-289, 1965.
27. Karam, J. H., Grodsky, G. N., and Fordsham, P. H.: Excessive insulin responses to glucose in obese subjects as measured by immunochemical assay. *Diabetes, 12*:197-204, 1963.
28. Perley, M. and Kipnis, D. M.: Differential plasma insulin responses to oral and infused glucose in normal weight and obese nondiabetic and diabetic subjects. *J Lab Clin Med, 66*:1009, 1965.
29. Perley, M. and Kipnis, D. M.: Plasma insulin responses to glucose and tolbutamide of normal weight and obese diabetic and nondiabetic subjects. *Diabetes, 15*:867-874, 1966.
30. Jorgensen, K. R.: Radioimmunoassay of insulin in plasma and urine in obese subjects and in diabetic patients. *Acta Endocrinol, 60*:719-736, 1969.
31. Beck, P., Koumans, J. H. T., Winterling, C. A., Stein, M. F., Daughaday, W. H., and Kipnis, D. M.: Studies of insulin and growth hormone secretion in human obesity. *J Lab Clin Med, 64*:654-667, 1964.
32. Porte, D., Graber, A. L., Kuzuya, T., and Williams, R. H.: The effect of epinephrine on immunoreactive insulin levels in man. *J Clin Invest, 45*:228-236, 1966.
33. Peake, G. T., McKeel, D. W., Mariz, I. K., Jarett, L., and Daughaday, W. H.: Insulin storage and release in rats bearing growth hormone secreting tumors. *Diabetes, 18*:619-624, 1969.
34. Malaisse, W. J., Malaisse-Lagae, F., King, S., and Wright, P. H.: Effect of growth hormone on insulin secretion. *Am J Physiol, 215*:423-428, 1968.
35. Fraser, R., Joplin, G. F., Opie, L. H., and Rabinowitz, D.: The augmented insulin tolerance test for detecting insulin resistance. *J Endocrinol, 25*:299-307, 1962.
36. Manougian, E., Pollycove, M., Linfoot, J. A., and Lawrence, J. H.: C[14] glucose kinetic studies in normal, diabetic, and acromegalic subjects. *J Nuclear Med, 5*:763-795, 1964.
37. Perley and Kipnis: Differential plasma insulin responses.

Chapter 5

SPORTS MEDICINE

Systematic physical conditioning pro-
grams undertaken by sedentary, middle-aged men[1] lead to an
improved physiologic status; not only is there an increased
subjective sense of well-being, there is also a beneficial
economy and efficiency of myocardial function and the oxygen
transport system. Young men[2, 3] participating in fitness programs are capable of developing some of the cardiorespiratory
characteristics of champion athletes. Running activities, calisthenics, and the use of special apparatus are traditional approaches to the development of fitness. They promote strength,
endurance, agility, coordination, and body control. When these
are undertaken in a gymnasium environment they frequently
are a social type of activity. Some find those exercises to be a
bore, and, after a brief warm-up, prefer competitive sports.

A variety of age groups participate in recreational sports. At
an age of about thirty-five years, the onset of middle age,
people begin to "slip," gain weight, lose agility, power, and
endurance. Reflexes as well as the general cardiorespiratory
status decrease. At that point in life, the individual is busy
supporting a family and the only time for exercise is at best
intermittent. At approximately the midpoint of life, recreational activities such as jogging, swimming, and tennis are
sought. The ageing process, especially when combined with
improper conditioning and warm-up, underlying systemic
problems, or preexisting defects, can cause injury-related problems.

Significant progress has been made in achieving a good understanding of the facets and techniques of many sports events.
Through that understanding, the mechanisms of injury occurring in sport activities are more readily determined, and therefore the diagnosis can be more exacting and the treatment more
effective. The following observations are based upon the per-

sonal experiences of Dr. James M. Glick, San Francisco, California, and provide a perspective of conditioning exercises and their attendant problems from an orthopedic point of view.

JOGGING

Jogging has become a desirable form of exercise. In 1969, injury data were obtained from two groups consisting of 120 middle-aged adults who participated voluntarily in an eleven-week jogging program.[4] One group was comprised of students and faculty members of the University of California at Berkeley and the other of persons in the San Francisco area. Two hundred and forty-one injuries of various types occurred. Forty-three percent were muscle strains or soreness, mostly of the calf muscle group. Twenty percent were joint sprains (soreness and swelling) of the knee and ankle. Eleven joggers were diagnosed as having "shin splints," i.e. pain in the lower leg about the shin. The most common cause is overuse resulting in muscle fatigue. There were two fatigue fractures, both in the distal shaft of the fibula near the ankle. The injuries were mild and none, including the fatigue fractures, caused permanent disability. It is felt that running-jogging is a relatively safe activity for the middle-aged adult.

TENNIS

A multitude of nagging injuries may occur from tennis. Shoulder pain occurs mainly during the serve and affects the rotator cuff muscles underneath the coracoacromial ligament. The biceps tendon may sometimes become irritated as it slides back and forth during the up and down motion of the arm.

Tennis elbow, by far, is the most common ailment in tennis. It is characterized by pain on the outer side of the elbow, which can be reproduced by palpation and shaking hands. Sometimes the inner side of the elbow can be affected. The exact cause and pathology of tennis elbow has yet to be determined. From a purely mechanical viewpoint this condition is caused by overuse of the muscles that stabilize the wrist and hand while gripping the racket. The extensor muscles originate at the lateral epicondyle on the outer side of the elbow. In order to grip the racket firmly, these muscles must work to their major capacity in order to stabilize the wrist. Therefore, they are contracted continuously while swinging a racket. When serving, these contracted muscles are stretched. The same is true on the backhand stroke. The same stress is not so prevalent on the forehand stroke. In a study of eighty-two tennis players, tennis elbow was attributed to the backhand four to one over the forehand and two to one over the serve. Three significant facts were present in 158 patients with tennis elbow: First, they were middle-aged, the average being forty-three years old; second, it usually started while gripping something, not only the tennis racket but a hammer or similar object; third, they were usually working with their hands in pronation (palm down), such as unscrewing a bottle top.

The wrist and hand are less frequently involved in tennis, but nevertheless can be a problem. Wrist sprains may occur if the wrist is jammed backwards while poorly hitting the ball. Hand problems usually consist of blisters and painful callouses, especially at the bases of the middle and ring fingers, where most of the gripping occurs.

Tennis leg is also a concern to some players. This condition consists of either a tear of the medial or inner belly of the gastrocnemius muscle in the lower leg, Achilles tendonitis, or most disabling, a tear of the Achilles tendon. The mechanism of injury is usually a foreful push-off of the foot with the toes firmly planted on the court. Initially it was felt that the sharp painful snap that occurs in the calf was due to a tear of the plantaris tendon, but actually it is the tearing of the medial belly of the gastrocnemius muscle.[5] This injury takes approximately six weeks to heal, but leaves the player without a disability. On the other hand, a ruptured Achilles tendon, no matter how treated, will usually leave the player with some restriction of ankle function.

GOLF

Golf has been a popular pastime sport for many years. Ten

years ago it was said that there were 4 million golfers. Now, there are reportedly 10 million golfers.[6] In the early years of golfing the courses were short, the shafts of the clubs were made out of wood, and the swing was mainly with the arm. Now, however, golf is a power game, as the courses are longer and the shafts of the clubs are metal. In order to get the maximum drive, the individual must use his entire body and this may initiate problems with the back, the hip, and even the elbow. The swing produces trunk hyperrotation in two directions, twisting of the leading hip and pronation forces on the lateral epicondyles of both elbows. These stresses after being repeated over and over can cause back strain, hip arthritis, and tennis elbow. Tennis elbow is not an uncommon condition in golfers.

SWIMMING

Swimming is an excellent therapeutic exercise. Although injuries are infrequent, shoulder pain and calf cramps may be troublesome conditions. In both the free style and butterfly strokes the supraspinatus tendon and the biceps tendon in the shoulder are exerted. As was discussed in the section on tennis, the rotator cuff passes over the humeral head to insert on the most superior portion of the humeral head. Likewise, the biceps tendon runs over the humeral head and attaches to the superior portion of the fossa of the shoulder. The repetitive underwater pulls and early arm recoveries of the free style and butterfly strokes may bring about early degenerative changes in these tendons.

Cramps are pain in the calf muscles that occur either during swimming or immediately after. The exact mechanism of swimmers' cramps is not known.

Diving injuries may be the most serious and disabling injuries that occur in swimming. When diving from a height, the neck should be extended so that the front part of the head strikes the water. The forces are then dissipated along the bony framework of the body. If the dive is made with the neck flexed, the top of the head strikes the water, resulting in forces that will hyperflex the neck which in turn may cause a fracture or dislocation[7] of the vertebrae.

HIKING

Foot pain and muscle soreness are the major problems in hiking. Frequently the hiker will acquire painful callosities and blisters on his feet. The muscles most commonly involved in walking are the gluteus maximus of the buttocks and the hamstrings in back of the thighs. These muscles decelerate or slow the leg during ambulation. Inman[8] has shown that more work is placed on the decelerators than on the accelerators while walking; those muscles therefore may show soreness.

BICYCLING

Despite the fact that on one occasion in the United States an attempt was made to ban bicycles as hazards, this form of transportation has grown steadily as an important physical activity. Overuse problems are most common in the quadriceps muscles in the thigh and patellar mechanisms. In addition, falling and striking other objects can cause more serious injuries.

The mechanism of injury to the quadricep and patellar mechanisms in bicycling is as follows: The quadricep muscles and the patella function maximally in pushing the pedal downward. When the knee is flexed just before the pedal is pushed downward, the patella is engaged tightly against the femur. As the knee is straightened to push the pedal downward, the quadricep muscle contracts strongly pressing the patella against its groove in the femur until the knee lacks about 30° from full extension. From this degree of extension to full extension the patella no longer engages in its groove. The constant action of the quadriceps muscle could eventually produce fatiguing pain and also softening of the undersurface of the patella. The latter is known as chondromalacia patella and is caused by repeated pressure of the patella against the femur. Therefore, the pain that commonly occurs from bicycling occurs around the upper or superior quarter of the kneecap (quadricep-tendonitis) or underneath the patella.

More serious injuries from falling or being struck by another vehicle consist of fractures, dislocations, and head injuries. In a review of bicycle injuries compiled in a Canadian community, 70 percent had serious head injuries. Twenty percent of these were due to a collision between the bicycle and an automobile.[9]

SKIING

The sport of skiing also produces a multitude of injuries, especially in the beginner and in the person who is not in good physical condition. The type of equipment has much to do with the type of injuries that occur. Low ski boots do not stabilize the ankle as well as the higher boots; therefore, one can expect more injuries about the ankle in the former. Fractures of the shafts of the leg bones (tibia and fibula) and injuries of the knee are more common when the high boot is worn. The high boot is being used more extensively by skiers today.

The most important piece of equipment in skiing is the release binding. No single binding has been found to be foolproof in the prevention of injuries. The skier should attempt to adjust the bindings as best as possible so that they will release when excessive forces are applied.

BALLET

The classical ballet dancer presents a special problem to the physician. Years of strenuous, daily activity which begins at an early age may produce alterations in the musculoskeletal system. Many women today are dancing in order to keep their figures trim, and some families have children participating in this most strenuous athletic endeavor.

As one might expect, dancers who dance on *pointe* develop changes in their feet, such as bunions and painful callosities. Because their choreography frequently calls for squats, the dancer will develop chondromalacia of the patella, such as the bicycle rider.

MANAGEMENT

No medical discussion is complete without statements about treatment which includes simple management which can be performed by the participants themselves. Rest is the major form of treatment. This does not mean that the activity has to be ceased altogether. Possibly only one part of the body can be placed at rest. For instance, an arm injury in a tennis player might restrict the playing of tennis, but the player may continue to keep in condition by running.

Shoulder pain is very difficult to treat. Shoulder pain is of three types. The first is pain only after activity; the second is nondisabling pain during and after activity; and the third is pain affecting performance. In the first, the shoulder should be used less during practice and ice applied for twenty to thirty minutes following exercise. In the nondisabling pain that occurs during and after activity, participants definitely will have to restrict their practice sessions. If they are swimmers, they should swim short distances, rather than long distances, at least until the pain subsides. If they are tennis players, serving will have to be restricted until match play commences. Ice again is a good form of treatment following activity. The person with disabling pain will have to rest completely for a period of time. A swimmer might have to change his or her event. Once the pain subsides, return to activity should be slow and gradual, possibly with the application of heat for fifteen minutes prior to participation, the application of counterirritants during performance, and then the application of ice following the event.

In most cases, jogging injuries are treated by the joggers themselves.[10] Muscle strains are treated by temporary rest, good running technique, and good running shoes. Joint sprains are probably best treated by attempting to run on a softer surface, the use of good running shoes and shoe pads. The fatigue fractures that were discussed were treated by temporary rest, either with or without a cast. It has been shown that the position of the pelvis is the key to postural control in running.[11] The jogger should attempt to run in a straight upright position so the spine is straight, and the pelvis rotated backwards. In this position the hips will remain flexed and externally rotated, therefore planting the foot onto the ground in a forward position. If on the other hand the runner is bent forward, the back becomes hyperextended, the pelvis rotates forward, and hip flexion and rotation are reduced, therefore the weight is placed on the ball of the foot and the foot is rotated in a flattened position. This places a great deal of stress on the muscles of the foot, can cause pressure on the ball of the foot, and can in general make running inefficient.

An inner wedge, in a running shoe, will sometimes help knee pain, especially the pain from chondromalacia of the patella.

The best treatment of tennis elbow is a cortisone injection, along with a period of rest. Bracing and exercises are useful in preventing further difficulties. The braces that are used should be lightweight and not restrict function. A simple strap around the bulk of the forearm is effective for tennis elbow; however, if the inner side of the elbow is affected, a brace with pads gripping the epicondyles is most effective. Stretching exercises, followed by wrist curls, using a 5 pound weight, are recommended exercises. Special wrist braces have been made to prevent dorsiflexion of the wrist. One-half inch heel pads are effective for treating Achilles tendonitis and injured calf muscles.

Hip and back pain, which occurs in golf, does not necessarily have to restrict the golfer entirely. The player might be able to continue practicing by using the old-fashioned arm swing with no body twist.

Swimmers' cramps are best treated by stretching the muscles. When hiking one should, of course, use proper boots; if blisters tend to occur, double socks, lubricants and pads can be used for protection.

Stretching sore muscles, the use of pads, and changing the position of the seat and pedals will frequently alleviate the aches and pains of the cyclist.

The ballet dancer will frequently wrap tape around blisters and just leave the tape in place until it finally falls off. The knee with chondromalacia of the patella should be strengthened by an isometric or straight-leg exercise. Placing a pillow underneath the knee and having the dancer push down on the pillow with the back of her knee is one way of performing this exercise.

THROUGH THE EYES OF THE SPECTATOR

Many sports enthusiasts wonder about injuries of the baseball player's arm and football player's knee. As might be expected, the baseball player places a great deal of stress on the arm. The elbow is as frequently involved as the shoulder. The mechanism of pitching places a stress on the inner side and on the outer side of the elbow. The repetitive throwing action produces traction injuries to the inner aspect of the elbow and traumatic interarticular injuries (arthritis) to the outer aspect of the elbow.

Children have a growth center on the inner aspect of the elbow that fuses to the humerus in the upper arm at the approximate age of fourteen. Irritation and pain at that point in the inner aspect of the elbow of youngsters is commonly known as "little league elbow." For the older athlete, changes in elasticity in the tendon of the flexor muscles in the inner elbow can produce a painful tendonitis.

The knees are the most vulnerable part of the football player's anatomy, and the shoe to surface interface is a very important factor in knee injuries. Artificial turf and the use of proper cleats have been reported to be helpful to some degree.

For an injury of the miniscii or semilunar cartilage to occur, the foot must be planted firmly on the ground. It usually occurs with the knee flexed at about 30 to 45° when the player attempts to change direction rapidly. If the normal twisting action is abruptly interrupted, the inner or outer cartilage will tear. Most commonly it is the inner cartilage.

A ligament injury of the knee occurs when a force is applied on the opposite side of the knee. Most commonly, the outer aspect of the leg is struck and the knee forced inward, causing a stretch or tear of the inner ligaments. The inner ligaments are the medial collateral or tibial collateral ligaments.

Meniscal tears do not heal and therefore the meniscus is removed if it is disabling. It does not have to be excised immediately after the injury. However, contrary to the miniscal injury, the completely torn ligament should be operated upon early to obtain the best results. Those individuals who sustain a completely torn ligament will most likely have surgery performed either immediately after an event or at least within the first five days following the injury.

REFERENCES

1. Hanson, J. S., Tabakin, B. S., Levy, A. M., and Nedde, W.: Long-term physical training and cardiovascular dynamics in middle-aged men. *Circulation, 38*:783-799, 1968.
2. Frick, M. H., Kontlinen, A., and Sarajas, H. S. S.: Effects of physical training on circulation at rest and during exercise. *Am J Cardiol, 12*:142-161, 1963.
3. Wang, Y., Shepherd, J. T., Marshall, R. J., Rowell, L., and Taylor, H. L.: Cardiac response to exercise in unconditioned young men and in athletes. (Abstract) *Circulation, 24*:1064, 1961.
4. Glick, J. M. and Katch, V. L.: Musculoskeletal injuries in jogging. *Arch Phys Med Rehabil, 51*:123-126, 1970.
5. Arner, C. O.: What is tennis leg? *Acta Chir Scand, 116*:73-75, 1958.
6. Stover, C. N.: Anatomical aspects of the upper extremity in the golf swing. Presented at the postgraduate course on Sports Medicine, American Academy of Orthopaedic Surgeons. Eugene, Oregon, 22 July 1974.
7. Schneider, R. C., Papo, M., and Soto-Alvarez, C.: The effects of chronic recurrent spinal trauma in high-diving. *J Bone Joint Surg, 44*:648-656, 1962.
8. Inman, V. T.: Conservation of energy in ambulation. *Arch Phys Med, 48*:484-488, 1967.
9. Guichon, D. M. P. and Myles, S. T.: Bicycle injuries: One-year sample in Calgary. *J Trauma, 15*:504-506, 1975.
10. Glick and Katch: Musculoskeletal injuries in jogging.
11. Slocum, D. B. and Bowerman, W.: Biomechanics of running. *Clin Orthop, 23*:39-45, 1962.

EPILOGUE

DURING the past thirty years, the United States population seems to have been faced with a physical fitness problem. Cureton et al.[1] summarized some of the findings regarding the fitness of young college-age men during the period 1940 to 1942. Some 20 to 25 percent of subjects tested could not chin themselves five times nor perform five pushups on parallel bars. Forty percent could not run a mile in seven minutes. Those results, along with additional criteria, led to a concern for the health and fitness future of young men. That concern was generalized to the belief that large numbers of young men were entering adult life unconditioned and unmotivated to do the physical labor necessary in life or to maintain physical fitness. This was believed to contribute significantly to high accident rates, rapid loss of health beyond the age of thirty, and widespread chronic disease. The American Medical Association[2] designated 1944 to 1945 as a "Physical Fitness Year" in the United States. In 1953,[3] impressive statistics were presented which related a low incidence of coronary heart disease and mortality to occupational physical activity. Mortality rate was considerably lower in laborers compared to light industry workers, for example. Men in physically active jobs had a lower incidence of coronary heart disease in middle age than men in physically inactive jobs. Importantly, the disease was not so severe in physically active workers with a lower early mortality rate. The International Study of Atherosclerosis[4] after reviewing the findings of approximately 23,000 autopsies collected from nineteen geographic and ethnic groups saw a sequential relationship between vascular fatty infiltration and coronary heart disease. The development of atherosclerosis was similar in all geographic locations studied, and race per se did not determine susceptibility to atherosclerosis. To the extent

97

that diet increases blood lipid level, it contributes to coronary heart disease. What is not clearly established is the extent that physical fitness protects against occlusive vascular disease. The results of exercise intervention studies have not been highly promising. Although the statistics cited by Morris et al.[5] show apparent protection in dock workers, coal miners, and laborers as compared to mechanics and typists, it is not clear that preventative exercise programs which improve muscular endurance are equivalent to a life of hard labor. Nor is it clear that a heavy industry worker would be judged to be highly fit on the basis of a cardiorespiratory test such as the maximum oxygen uptake.

Obesity poses a significant health problem in that susceptibility to chronic disease is enhanced and length of life is decreased.[6] The syndrome is related to overeating and sedentary living. There may be specific abnormalities in endocrine function, particularly in the pancreas, adrenal, and thyroid, although the metabolic responses during exercise, and carbohydrate and fat metabolism are not consistently different from the expected normal range. Because of body weight, the metabolic cost of exercise is high, and left ventricular hypertrophy is a common finding in autopsies of obese people. Control of appetite is the best treatment. In the event that caloric intake cannot be reduced sufficiently, obesity can only be prevented by an increase in physical activity. Further studies are required to elaborate the trends of weight loss in relationship to degree of caloric deficit. Reports of greater fat losses on moderately restricted diets (1000 to 1500 kg Cal/day) than during total food deprivation need further development and amplification.

The effect of withdrawal or deficiency of the major nutrients on performance is moderately well understood both in terms of the time history of deterioration as well as the specific systems affected. Water, calories, and salt are principal requirements, and their impact on performance is known with sufficient confidence to prescribe a variety of menus and dietaries including those for planned minimal feeding concepts. The effect of deprivation of the trace elements and lesser understood micronutrients on performance is unknown and the real nutritional defects associated with those deficiencies in man are yet to be discovered. The characteristics of "subclinical" nutritional deficiencies are highly controversial and have led to a certain amount of faddism in associating performance capability with special food supplements.

On the other hand, competition class athletes do benefit from the intake of high carbohydrate diets for several days prior to a contest, and thus they show improvement by manipulation of calorie source.

The environment imposes particular requirements, especially conditions which promote body water and salt loss. Increased food energy requirements in a cold environment[7] are related to shivering, heat exchange with the environment, and the encumbrance of environmental protective clothing and equipment on walking activities. Special conditions such as those cited for space exploration may require additional electrolyte supplementation.

Although there exists a large number of documented gross responses to exercise and diet, the specific details which give rise to decrements in performance as a result of dietary deprivations are not known. For example, why does the heart rate during work increase after one day of fasting? Is the increased heart rate mediated by the nervous system or by other factors? Why is there a decrement in the ability to perform short bouts of exhaustive work under the same conditions? That work is performed by muscles which have a relatively high capacity for anaerobic metabolism. Is the limitation at the cellular level or related to possible variations in blood transport? Those are the details required to properly elucidate the specific mechanisms involved. Answers to those questions probably will be developed within an interdisciplinary research environment in which there will be a continuing need for better research methods and more adequate conceptual systems within disciplines. The discussions in Chapters 3 and 4 of the involvement of hormones in exercise, as well as in obesity, show how really "soft" the data base is. For example, if the obese have hypersecretory insulin responses, the expectation is that the level of plasma free fatty acid would be lower than normal. However, apparently that is not the case; hence, the evaluation is clouded by either problems of methodology or the involvement of a multiplicity of factors. Solid progress will be made through a pooling and sharing of information and methodologies. There is still room for intuitive approaches in conceptualizing problems.

It would appear to be important to learn and enjoy activities that involve locomotion and the movement of the body and which can be accommodated within a life style. That this area is of much more than academic interest is attested to by the rapidly expanding development of exercise programs with purported prophylactic and therapeutic cardiovascular effects. It is generally understood that an increased level of physical fitness enables the individual to meet physical demands with the least strain of functional effort and with lesser consequences of physical fatigue. The risks involved in most exercises are quite low. Supervised exercise tests utilized as diagnostic cardiovascular procedures are also low risk,[7] and increase, by a considerable factor, the yield of information from the electrocardiogram.

Participation in sports and exercises should be with the individuals' knowledge of their own limitations, an understanding of safety factors where appropriate, and by exercising common sense to restrict injuries.

During the past fifteen years there have been relatively few advances in gaining newer insights into the influence of diet per se on physical work capacity. Our knowledge today is based more or less on a data base available in 1958 to 1960. What remains to be developed in quite some detail is the cellular biochemical basis for variations and decrements in performance. However, at the present there seems to be relatively little interest in that approach.

The neuroendocrine responses during exercise and in grossly altered nutritional states such as obesity have been researched in considerable detail with emphasis on insulin-growth hormone mechanisms and carbohydrate/fat metabolism. Insulin does not play a significant role in the enhancement of carbohydrate metabolism during exercise, but is probably involved in the development of obesity. However, pieces of the puzzle are still missing and a comprehensive description of the causalities of obesity is not yet possible.

Studies of exercise intervention for ischemic heart disease have probably moved into a second phase of investigation. Now there is some appreciation for the numbers, health status (risk factors), and experiment design requirements for future studies. Those studies which were undertaken to relate diet to the pathogenesis of atherosclerosis have been somewhat derelict in not providing good data on nutrient intake determined by direct food analysis. Recognizing that it would be quite difficult to assess the food intake in a large population tested, still if it is one of the experimental variables, the diet should be recognized and understood.

In conclusion, there are still considerable gaps of knowledge in the understanding of the relationships between diet, fitness, and performance and many intriguing areas of investigation which can contribute to a coherent picture of those interactions. The interested reader is urged to review some of the older literature cited in this monograph in order to gain a greater perspective of the relationships between diet and fitness.

REFERENCES

1. Cureton, T. K., Huffman, W. J., Welser, L., Kireilis, R. W., and Latham, D. E.: Endurance of young men. Analysis of endurance exercises and methods of evaluating motor fitness. Monograph, *Society for Research in Child Development, 10*, No. 1, Serial No. 40, 284 pp., National Research Council, Washington, D.C., 1945.
2. Fishbein, M.: Physical fitness program. *JAMA, 125*:840-851, 1944.
3. Morris, J. N., Heady, J. A., Raffle, P. A. B., Roberts, C. B., and Parks, J. W.: Coronary heart disease and physical activity of work. *Lancet, 2*:1111-1120, 1953.
4. McGill, H. C.: The geographic pathology of atherosclerosis. *J Lab Invest, 18*:463-653, 1968.
5. Morris et al.: Coronary heart disease and physical activity of work.
6. U.S. Public Health Service, Division of Chronic Diseases. Obesity and health: A source book of current information for professional health personnel. Washington, D.C., U.S. Government Printing Office, 1966.
7. Johnson, R. E., and Kark, R. M.: Environment and food intake in man. *Science, 105*:378, 1947.
8. Rochmis, P. and Blackburn, H.: Exercise tests. A survey of procedures, safety, and litigation experience in approximately 170,000 tests. *JAMA, 217*:1061-1066, 1971.

AUTHOR INDEX

103

SUBJECT INDEX

A

Acetone, 27
Achilles tendonitis, 88
Acid sodium phosphate (NaH_2PO_4), 42
Acidosis, 7, 13, 22, 24, 33, 57
Acromegalics, 83
Adipose tissue, 32, 55, 83
  free fatty acid release, 58
  lipid, conversion of glucose to, 60
Adrenalcortical hormones, 26
Aerobic capacity, 41
  maximal, 30
Adlosterone, 43
Amino acids, 19
  imbalance, vii
Anaerobic metabolic capacity, 23, 24
Angina, 8
Antidiuretic hormone, 43
Arrhythmias, cardiac, 43
Arthritis, 94
  hip, 89
Ascorbic acid (see Vitamin C)
Atherosclerosis, vi, 8
  coronary, 62
Atrophy, muscle disuse, 43

B

Back pain, 93
Back strain, 89
Ballet, 91
Basal metabolic rate, lowering of, vii
Beri-beri, 13
Bicarbonate, 21
Biceps tendon, 87, 89
Bicycle ergometer, 57
Bicycling, 90-91
Blood pressure, 23
  decreases, 8
Blood sugar, 7, 8, 18, 24, 36, 38

  low, 21
  obesity, effect of, 60
Bone meal, 8

C

Calcium, 11, 40
Calf, cramps of, 89
Calisthenics, 30
Calorie
  deficiency, vii
  imbalance, 16
  requirements, 29
Carbohydrates, 3, 24, 27, 38, 39, 58
  deficiency, 13
  diets, high, 37
  intake, lowered, 25
  metabolism, 9
  triglycerides, relation to, 62
Cardiorespiratory system
  deconditioning, 21
  overweight, effect of, 52
Cardiovascular system
  disease, 3
  overweight, effect of, 52
  reserve, 24
  semistarvation, in, 16
  starvation, in, 16
Casein, 27
Chilomicrons, 82
Chloride, 20
Cholesterol, vi, 40, 41, 62
Chondromalacia patella, 90, 91, 93
Climatic stress, 11
Coordination, loss of, 16, 24
Coracoacromial ligament, 87
Cortisone injection, 93
Cramps, 93
  calf, 89
  heat, 13

Tendonitis, 94
 achilles, 88
Tennis, 87
Tennis elbow, 87-88, 89, 93
Tennis leg, 88
Thiamine, 7, 11
Thiocyanate space, water shifts in, 20
Thyroid, atrophy of, 18
Tibia, 91
Tolbutamide, 82
Treadmill walking, 24, 25, 30, 32, 37, 40, 50, 57, 63
Triglycerides, vi, 8
 weight, body, relationship to, 62

U

Undernutrition, viii
 chronic, 7, 20
Urates, 19
Urea, blood, 19
Uric acid, 19
Urine, 24
 volume, 26

V

Vitamin
 A, 14
  deficiency, 13
 B complex, 7, 8
  deficiency, 13
 C, vi, 8, 11, 21
  deficiency, 13
 E, 8
 starvation, deficiency during, 21
Vomiting, 24

W

Water, 12, 26
 balance, 7
 conservation, 24
 deficiency, 13, 14
 extracellular space, 20, 24
 loss, 43
  evaporative, 25
 requirements, minimum, 24-25
 weight loss, shifts with, 20
Weight loss, 16-18
Work, calorie expenditures, 30
Wrist sprains, 88